Always In Touch

Always In Touch

A Practical Guide to Ubiquitous Computing

by
David G. Brown

WAKE FOREST UNIVERSITY PRESS
– SCIENTIFIC DIVISION –
WINSTON-SALEM

ISBN: 0-9644070-2-7

Ubiquitous

U·biq·ui·tous (yo͞o bik´wi təs), *adj.* existing or being
everywhere, esp. at the same time; omnipresent.
u·biq´ui·tous·ly *adv.* – **u·biq´ui·tous·ness**, *n.*

CONTENTS

PREFACE

"The intention of this slim volume is to identify key concepts and strategies that are critical to efficient computing and communications."

As professor, president, and provost in both the public and private sector, in both colleges and universities, I have personally struggled with decisions about "how best to teach" and "where most efficiently to invest in technology." Since 1996 when Wake Forest University (where I served as Professor of Economics and Provost) started providing powerful laptop computers to all students and faculty, I have spoken (mainly at professional meetings) with at least 1,200 presidents and provosts, helped host over 300 colleges and universities on our campus, run several dozen workshops for teams of decision makers, consulted with dozens of schools and communities, and regularly used technology in my own teaching. From these experiences emerge a crisp concept of the key issues involved and the decisions that face each college and university in the next five years.

Since January 1998 when special arrangements were made to cover my other provost responsibilities at Wake Forest, I have devoted full time (now as Vice President and Dean of the Wake Forest University International Center for Computer Enhanced Learning) to coaching others on how to maximize their computer investment decisions and, most of all, their teaching (and research) effectiveness.

In a companion volume, *Learning Enhanced by Computers: A Case Study of Wake Forest University*, "the Wake Forest Story" is told in more detail. In that edited volume, the intention is for the experience at Wake Forest University to be a catalyst for thinking about the role of technology in other institutions. Each group comes to the technology decision with differing emphases, differing champions, differing "neighborhood" resources, differing computing legacies, differing financial resources, differing governance structures, differing user groups (e.g. part-time and full-time students), differing scale, differing philosophies and subject matters, differing market opportunities, and differing propensities to risk. No single plan fits all!

The intention of this slim volume is to help professors and presidents, deans and faculty, students and trustees, donors and legislators, school teachers and superintendents, mayors and city managers, community and economic developers, chief information officers and course designers identify key concepts and strategies that are critical to establishing and maintaining an efficient computing and communications environment. These should be broadly and clearly articulated throughout the implementing community so that its many decision makers can contribute to a coherent, effective and efficient system.

For educating me to the potential of computers, I want to thank my students as well as John Anderson, Jay Dominick, Rick Matthews, and Jennifer Burg. For adding to the list of "lessons learned," my gratitude goes to David Blyler, Rhoda Channing, Lynda Goff—all of Wake Forest—plus Mark Resmer (Sonoma State), Dan Updegrove (Yale), Diana Oblinger (IBM), Ray Brown (Mayville State and Valley City State), Larry Bryant (US Air Force Academy), and Irving Blythe (Virginia). Aggressive editing by Cornelia Wright added greatly to readability, and I thank her for it. Thanks also to Janet Bright and Janice Schuyler who shepherded the manuscript to publication.

David G. Brown
Winston-Salem, NC
Brown@wfu.edu
January, 1999

Always In Touch

A Practical Guide to Ubiquitous Computing

CHAPTER I

INTRODUCTION

*". . . computers allow a single individual to establish
and maintain connections with more subgroups,
with more people, from more places, with greater intensity
for longer periods of time."*

The central thesis of this book is that computers allow a single individual to establish and maintain connections in more subgroups, with more people, from more places, with greater intensity for longer periods of time. The connecting power of the computer, not fancy PowerPoint presentations or more sophisticated statistical analyses, has raised the ceiling on how far we can go passing along accumulated wisdom.

The revolution is about connectedness. There are many other ways to use computers. These are not the concern of this book. Our focus is upon communication, connections, community. This book is about how a college, a school system, even a whole community can build a stronger infrastructure for communication.

Most references are to the experience of colleges. For now, they are our most wired sub-communities. A college campus is a self-contained laboratory to explore the potential of computers for enhancing communication. In time, as other communities increase their access to technology and as computer-literate students move on after graduation, school systems and entire communities will be able to put systems in place that ultimately will transform the quality of human interactions. This book is about using the computer to enhance communication.

Each chapter is written to stand alone, so time-deprived folks can skip immediately to the topics of greatest interest. First we retrace some of the most basic reasons communities are investing so heavily in computers (Chapter 2). After describing 20 guiding metaphors (Chapter 3), a dozen basic issues that must be resolved in every strategic plan for computing are outlined (Chapter 4). Following a description of the 10 phases (e.g., deciding, implementing, assessing), strategies for building consensus are detailed (Chapter 5). A discussion of faculty culture and faculty development strategies (Chapter 6) is followed by a list of ways computers are being used to pursue the 7 principles of good teaching (Chapter 7). Chapter 8 focuses upon "lessons learned."

The final chapter looks to the future. How will the computer-driven paradigm shift become ubiquitous throughout our most effective schools systems and communities, and how will computers change higher education? My hope and expectation is that each reader of this volume will add to, even critique, the existing chapter by serving as a voluntary editor. My intention is to update this final chapter, with appropriate credits, on the basis of your input. During the first year of publication, I expect to edit the chapter six times per year. So, please read this volume with the expectation that you too should contribute to our ever-growing body of knowledge on these important matters.

CHAPTER 2

THE COMPELLING CASE FOR UNIVERSAL COMPUTERS

*"The computer is the new 'great enabler' of community
building, collaborating, teaming, sharing, education."*

Communication! Communication! Communication!

The marketplace has already answered the question, "Are computers useful and wanted?" Computers are here and increasing! Students without computers want them. Students with them, use them. There is virtually no community that has adopted a computer-based communication network and then chosen to abandon it.

Why has the adoption of, and longing for, computers-for-communication become so pervasive so quickly? At its core, education is passing information from teacher to learner, from one generation to another. Teaching and learning centrally involves communicating. By book and movie, telephone and lecture, discussion and office conference, apprenticing and mentoring—knowledge is passed from one generation to another.

In *Bowling Alone*, Robert Putnam documents the worldwide phenomenon of withdrawal from group activity in the twentieth century. "The trend has been from participating to spectating, from choral societies to individual piano lessons, from large political parties to special-interest groups, from bowling leagues to individual bowling sessions." Putnam goes on to say, "The computer is enabling a rebirth of community and will likely reverse the trend toward bowling alone." Suddenly, communities can be built and sustained without regard to geographic distance and without the necessity of "simultaneous presence."

Like textbooks and the printing press before them, computers magnify our options for communicating in two fundamental ways: (1) by giving a single individual more access to more information in more useful formats in less time at less cost, and (2) by allowing a single individual to be more active in more communities with more people, and to sustain those commitments over more miles and more years. Computers allow an individual to become and stay more connected to more information and more people, at less cost. More community! More connectedness! The paradigm shift involved is enormous.

What is so special about the computer is that it combines the function of several existing media interactively. It can function like a book or library, providing access to information, while it simultaneously functions like a telephone, enabling two-way communication. It takes a quantum leap beyond these media in the quantity of information it can store and provide, and in the level of connectedness it can sustain. This interactive "innovation" is the most comprehensive breakthrough in both the storage and transmission of knowledge in this century. It changes all possibilities!

The computer is the new "great enabler" of community building, collaborating, teaming, sharing, educating. The new conversations and the new communities are a hybrid of face-to-face contact and of keeping in touch "virtually." Much like church and synagogue groups, the community gathers "once a week" while contact is sustained between meetings through largely independent pursuits within the parameters of shared values.

Nine Other Reasons to Adopt Universal Computers

The single, overwhelming reason computers are being adopted everywhere is their impact upon connectedness. Listed below are nine "sub-reasons" why computers are so important in organizations that emphasize community.

1. Computers vs. Phones

Computers increase the quality, the character, the consistency, and the continuity of conversation. This new communication device, "a thousand times" more powerful than a telephone and its answering machine, carries still and motion video, a broad range of textual materials, and hyperlinks to elaborations—this in addition to audio. Messages are conveniently sent from one individual to a group. Delivery times can be specified. "Conversations" on a specific topic can be threaded, even though the elements of a particular conversation are not contiguous. Messages can be regularly sorted by sender, by recipient, by topic, by date. Archived dialogue can be selectively retrieved by various search engines.

2. Collaborative Learning

Through enhanced communities, computers enrich collaborative learning. How blessed we are when we can walk through life accompanied by a diversity of people who are willing to share their enthusiasms, their passions, their perspectives, and their knowledge with us. This is the strength of collaborative learning, a learning style greatly facilitated by the computer.

Picture a person walking alone along a rural road. He or she spots a piece of folded paper and picks it up. The folds are neat. Both sides are blank, without text or picture. Our solitary hiker stands contemplating the new find. Now, think of this person accompanied by a child who playfully recognizes the folded piece of paper as an airplane, by an artist who carefully unfolds the paper and notes contour and shape, by a paper manufacturer who evaluates grade and texture and gloss and color, and by the neatnik who must pick up the paper as trash. By collaborating, by sharing perspectives, much is to be gained. Because the computer enables a single individual to be more intensely involved in more communities, the potential for collaboration is vastly increased.

3. Level Playing Field

Today's reality is that about 30 percent of all households and 50 percent of all college students have 24-hour access to the Internet. With such access comes privilege such as timely updates, immediate notifications, search engines for relevant social services, easier collaborations, membership in more communities, and knowledge and entertainment of all types. With knowledge comes power. As we build toward a society of openly accessible data bases, the disparity between those who have access and those who do not will grow. Such inequities are simply unacceptable. In colleges, it is unacceptable to teach on the assumption that all students have textbooks when some cannot gain access to one. It is unacceptable for only some students to have a key to the library. Now that computer data bases have become so important and continuous communication with professors and fellow students has become so prevalent, it is no longer fair to deny some students access to computers when they are being measured against other students who have computers. Since it is neither wise nor politic to prohibit computer use by the "have's," the only way to achieve equity is to provide computers for the "have nots." Until such provisions are in place, we can expect that faculty and community adoption of truly new modes of instruction and governance will not evolve, not until computers are universally accessible.

Public computer laboratories are more economically feasible and a reasonable alternative to personal ownership, but like textbooks on reserve reading in the campus library, and time-share condominiums; public computer labs are not adequate substitutes for personal "anytime, anywhere" ownership.

Desktop computers are a more economically feasible and a reasonable alternative to laptop ownership—but like refrigerators and bedroom furniture and mobile phones, important flexibility is gained when computers can be "on site" whenever needed. This characteristic is especially important in the sciences where in-class use of the computer is often essential, in study-abroad programs so that students may stay in touch with the main campus, and with part-time students who have a difficulty reaching the laboratory during open hours and at times surrounding a class session.

4. Dominant Use After Graduation

One of our goals is to graduate students with ability and self-confidence. By providing computers and software that students are most likely to meet upon graduation, we should be able to enhance both qualities. Wake Forest's adoption of the Microsoft operating system, Lotus GroupWare, Microsoft Office, Netscape Browser, and Wintel-based IBM ThinkPad stems from a desire to graduate students who have the best chance of feeling good about themselves in a new environment, something that can be enhanced by knowing you know the computer system.

5. The Market Demand

One of the most dramatic benefits of providing computers to all students, according to reports from colleges that have implemented ubiquitous computing, is the size and quality of applicants for vacant faculty positions. Evidently, younger faculty have themselves become "addicted" to the availability of the computer and are reluctant to teach in environments where their students don't have that same advantage. As K-12 systems adopt computers, we can expect similar impacts upon faculty requirement. Also, as entire communities adopt ubiquitous computing strategies, we can expect site selection teams not only to use the "extent of computerization" both as another measure of K-12 effectiveness and as an index of the "quality of life" in the community-as-a-whole. Prospective college students, K-12 parents, and "business relocation specialists" are being influenced not only by information they collect via the internet but also by the extent of computerization in the communities they are considering joining.

6. Marketable Difference

Having something specific (a new computer with you all the time) to differentiate our program has proven to be very attractive not only to incoming students but also their tuition-paying parents. By increasing the flow of student applications, it is possible to remain discriminating in the selection of a new class.

7. Computers Throughout the Day and Throughout Life

One of the characteristics of computers is that they allow an individual to remain a more active member of more communities for more years. For colleges this can mean a very active relationship with alumni, fuller offerings of continuing education courses, greater use of alumni as "guest commentators" and job contacts for graduating seniors, and an ability to update information that may have changed since students took a particular course. Students, who come to know a college's computer system during their four years on campus, will be inclined to continue accessing information and friends through that system; and they will be disadvantaged if this means of access is no longer available to them.

To the K-12 student, continuous access may relate to access at school and similar access when doing homework at night. To the community member, continuous access may mean access at work and at home.

The advantage of ubiquitous computing systems designed for continuous access is the dependability and continuity of communication.

8. Customization

I frequently tell the story of talking to the provost at a large university where organic chemistry is taught to classes of 1,200 students, this compared to about 25 student classes at a small liberal-arts college. At the large university, students working through homework assignments e-mailed their individual questions to a hierarchy of undergraduate chemistry majors, beginning graduate students, all-but-dissertation students, assistant professors, and ultimately the senior professor who gave the lecture in the morning. At each level, an individual answer, which would often include suggested readings in an alternative textbook, was given to the student and unanswered questions were referred up the hierarchy. In this way, through technology, the 1200-student class became more customized than the 25-student class!

Whether it's greeting cards designed and printed while we wait, high quality windows in the exact size we want, new automobiles finished to our specifications, or mail-order catalogs sent to a list tailored to customers' zip-codes; massive increases in choices we have mean that customization is increasingly expected and demanded in college educations, in the developmental opportunities we design for K-12 students, and in the services we provide throughout our communities. New opportunities for customization will soon become mandatory levels against which adequate performance will be measured.

9. Access to Scholarship

Increasingly, the scholarly discourse to which all students need access will be carried out in electronic databases. Printed books and journals are likely to persevere for reasons of convenience and archiving, at least until computers achieve the portability of books and migrating old data to new systems becomes less difficult and more certain. Most scholarly materials will, however, be more readily and fully accessible through computers and the Internet. Most "textbooks" will be supplemented by CD-ROMs.

Citations are more meaningful when hyperlinked to the cited source. Concepts are better understood when hyperlinked to fuller explanations. Relevant research is more likely to be uncovered when searches can be pursued by multiple means (e.g. date, author, location, key word, a phrase, and so on).

Electronic databases may gather in a single location not only text but also audio and video materials. Instructions may be imbedded in the materials that automatically update data that are actively managed at another Internet site. Errata can be immediately linked to original manuscripts.

Font size and style, even language, can be customized to the individual reader. New information on specified topics can automatically be pushed to the scholar's desktop.

Properly construction electronic databases allow the "reader" to manipulate (e.g., to rotate a sculpture), to interact (e.g., with the author), and to collaborate asynchronously (as well as synchronously).

The new economics of publishing and distribution will undoubtedly mean that some scholarly information will be more affordable when delivered electronically and when made available for a specific time interval.

Because most scholars cherish the widest distribution of their ideas, the Internet has already become a major highway for exchange.

CHAPTER 3

METAPHORS FOR MAKING DECISIONS

"By thinking metaphorically about computers, we can free up our minds to imagine new ways to teach and learn."

Decisions around how to implement computers for communication are best made with two things in mind: the objectives of the technology plan and a contextual understanding of current technology and where's its likely headed. The context suggests what's possible. The objectives suggest what's best.

Most of us agree that the computer revolution is taking us in directions we never anticipated and leading us to think in terms of models we never envisioned, a process as fascinating as it is terrifying. One Web page developer describes this as the state of *vuja de*, "the strange feeling we've never been here before." As we pick our ways through the theories and constructs, metaphors can help us free up our minds to imagine ways of applying these new practices. By relating the strange to the familiar, by linking predictions with current practice; the unfamiliar territory of computers can take shape in the minds of decision-makers. By thinking metaphorically about computers and their use for study and research, consistency and predictability can be lent to focussed judgements. In this spirit, a dozen metaphors are cited .

• Automobile in the Jungle

Futurist George Gilder asks us to image a person not previously exposed to the modern world struggling through jungle underbrush and happening upon a 1990s automobile that had been dropped by helicopter into a grove of trees. Curiosity might well yield observations such as "this is a wonderful place to sit down," "in this chamber climate can be controlled and insects cannot reach me," "the radio brings music and voice in many variations," "the gasoline tank is a generous decanter for liquids of all types," "the trunk is a watertight storage bin," and "this chamber can be reoriented, facing into the sun or away from it."

Now think about this same discovery taking place, but this time next to a highway with automobiles whizzing by. With a network of roads the automobile takes on real meaning, as a means of getting from one place to another. Without a highway network the automobile is limited, underutilized, and misunderstood.

The computer standing alone is much like the automobile in the jungle. The real magic doesn't occur until networks enable freestanding computers to connect with each other. The true revolution in technology is the combination of the computers and the networks: one without the other is of little significance. When shaping a local system, it is important to plan not only for destination computers (e.g., laptops) but also for network enablers (servers) and access ramps (transmission lines) to other clusters.

• 1000 Times More Powerful Telephones

Like the telephone, the computer is most significantly for communicating. In an education context, the computer revolution is about communication, about group connectedness, about community. The major benefits from computers cannot be realized until an entire community, each of its members, joins in much in the same way that all folks had to be accessible by phone before its full meaning became apparent.

When only a few people owned telephones and no one had an answering machine, use was limited to special occasions. Now that virtually everyone can be reached by phone, even when not present, the phone is becoming a standard medium for announcing meetings and sharing messages. As computers become equally ubiquitous, we can expect their use as a basic communication medium to soar in as yet unimagined ways.

The computer's capacity to accommodate communication is much, much more flexible, diverse, and rich than the telephone. The computer can manage threaded conversations, file and search-retrieve messages, support interactive video conferencing, send simultaneous messages to groups, forward messages selectively, give selective access to files of messages, accommodate text with sound and video, provide standardized formats and forms, and do everything at a very low cost that now is not metered by distance.

• Rural Electrification

In the United States, there came a time about seventy years ago when products and policies presumed that all citizens had access to basic electricity. Electrical service became a right, no longer merely a privilege. Federal legislation followed that assured electricity even in the nation's more remote communities. Even though the cost of extending electricity to remote areas was quite high, it was done because it was essential and fair.

Like electricity, computers are becoming ubiquitous and essential. Equal access to government documents, to news and entertainment, to banks and (perhaps) voting will eventually require "rural computerization." The basic computer infrastructure will necessarily be accessible to all citizens. Using the computer will become a base skill, just as turning a light switch is a possibility in every household in the United States today.

• Key to the Library

Colleges would not think of locking some students out of their library and laboratories while continuing to give other students unlimited access. This is a matter of equity and justice. Right now, however, except at colleges that insist on universal computers, there is a gap between those students who own computers (about 50 percent in most colleges and well above 50 percent in many) and those who do not. It is as if some students have keys to the library and others don't.

Such unbalanced access to the basic infrastructure is not fair and will not be tolerated for long. As computers become more and more useful and ubiquitous, the consequences of the gap will escalate. Since it is not realistic to prohibit students who own computers from bringing them to college, equity considerations mandate that students who come to college without their own computers be provided equal access.

As computers become ubiquitous in all aspects of life, schools and communities will face the same dilemma now best seen in colleges. Each aspect of our communities will have its "key to the library" that must not be denied any citizen.

• Cost of the Library

Originally libraries were personal collections. Neither colleges nor towns had them. Over time, however, Benjamin Franklin's idea of the public library took hold. Today, few communities in the United States are without them.

In colleges, the library has become equally expected and routine. At first, each new expenditure for acquisitions or service was marginal to the budget and required separate justification. By now, there have developed standard guidelines concerning library expenditures. When counting space and staff and acquisitions, libraries are now expected to cost about 6 percent of the total educational and general budgets (smaller colleges must spend more, and larger colleges can escape with slightly lower percentages).

A useful concept in contemplating the eventual cost of computing systems in most college and universities is this same six percent. By focusing on six percent as a goal, realistic multi-year planning can shape a system that is scaled to fit.

• General Contractor

When building a new structure (e.g., a house) one strategy is to hire a general contractor who in turn coordinates subcontractors to do the plumbing, heating and air conditioning, electricity, roofing, etc. An alternate strategy is to forgo hiring a general contractor and to do all the subcontracting yourself.

There are clear advantages to both systems. The experienced general contractor knows the strengths and weaknesses of potential subcontractors and the sequence of projects and the lead times to get materials to the job. The general contractor accepts full responsibility for the coordination of a complex project, and often (due to volume) has leverage with subcontractors. On the other hand, the subcontracting strategy is often less expensive. The owner has more discrete control of each aspect of the project. The owner can at each phase ask for competitive bids and make personal choices among those received.

Most large organizations, and many people having personal houses built for them, settle on the general contractor strategy. In the world of computers, however, most institutions are their own subcontractors. They go out and buy servers, then separately desktops or laptops, then separately software systems. They accept responsibility for coordinating the various vendors.

Worthy of consideration is the identification of a single primary vendor, or cluster of long-term vendors, who will accept responsibility for coordination and compatibility. The primary vendor in this model must offer a broad spectrum of services, and therefore can be expected to meet most challenges.

• Students as Nomads

Throughout the world, college students are a privileged class of nomads. When you ask their address, they respond: "Do you mean my campus address, my home address, and where I'll be this summer?" Throughout the year they sleep in many different beds. Few have offices. Many spend semesters abroad.

When college students complete their studies, rarely do they stay in place. The infrastructure available to them when studying must, however, somehow continue to be available to them after graduation—for their thinking processes have been molded with the presumption that the tools available in college will continue to be available throughout life.

Computer strategies must be designed to realistically accommodate the living patterns of all those who use computers, whether students or pupils or citizens.

• A New Set of Garden Tools

In the last 30 years there has never been a time when so many faculty, and so many disciplinary professional associations, have been thinking so much about teaching—what's taught, what should be taught, and how it is best taught. The value systems of the profession have swung toward rewarding effort and success in teaching.

The new emphasis upon teaching should not be a surprise. Of foremost concern to faculty has always been how students learn. Virtually all members of our profession are open to new ideas and are quick to consider the usefulness of new methodologies as soon as they appear. The apparent indifference to teaching that set over the profession for the past 50 years has been more the result of "more of the same old" and of the absence of any major innovation opportunities.

With computerization has come the opportunity to use very different teaching methods. Degrees have freedom have been radically expanded. In such an environment it makes sense that faculty would take the time to rethink what they are doing and why, to consider all ways they might improve (including non-technological ways), and then to fashion new strategies that mix in what they find to be the most successful new tools.

Suddenly, the profession has received a massive shipment of new gardening tools. Being a curious lot, and wanting the best growth possible, professors everywhere are experimenting. If we use this new tool in this way on this type of plant, will growth be advanced? Coupled with adventuresome curiosity is a conservative concern that experiments be structured in a way that no crop is killed off. In the end, we can expect that the old reliable tools will be the mainstays of the garden but that the most successful gardeners will be selectively using the new tools.

Faculty development programs should be based upon the assumption that faculties will be pushing Information Systems (IS) Departments to support course redesign, and that the challenge of IS departments is not to motivate faculty but rather to keep up with faculty who are already being motivated by their peers and their profession. It is neither necessary nor wise to mandate the adoption in all disciplines by all professors for all students the use of still yet barely tested techniques. The mores of the professions will push adoption forward as fast as is desirable. We are a profession of curious gardeners and love experimenting with new tools.

• House Calls and Outpatient Clinics

In medicine, individual consultations are the norm. Occasionally, we may attend a wellness clinic. Often we'll read on our own about a health issue that impacts us. We are, however, unlikely to attend a general orientation about arthritis until we are diagnosed with it. Medical information is sought out on a "need to know" and individual basis.

When we visit the doctor it is usually one on one. If our health seems linked to our work or home environment, usually a medical specialist (not always the doctor) will even make a house call.

The paradigm for computer help desks and for computer training follows this same model. Advice must be individual provided, just in time when there is a perceived need to know. A strong computer support system offers opportunities for call in advice, for training on demand, for referral to specialists, for experts in diagnosis, and when necessary even house calls (less important when the "patient's" computer is portable). Staffing and policies wisely follow the medical model.

• Learning a Second Language by Immersion

The easiest way to pick up a second language is to live in that culture. Children learn basic language by being around it, by being in a society where everyone speaks it.

Increasingly, younger generations are acquiring computer skills in the same way. They are surrounded by peers using computers and somehow, perhaps by osmosis, they pick up the skills. One of the great advantages of standardized ubiquitous computing is that everyone in the community is not only surrounded by people using computers, but also that they are all using the same programs on similar computers. In such an environment very little special instruction is required. Users acquire needed knowledge simply by frequent association with others who already have it.

In colleges and communities where dollars are scarce, depending upon learning by immersion is a valuable strategy. While backup systems need to exist, the main burden of training can take place naturally.

• State Religion

Many countries harbor a close relationship between the governmental state and a particular religion. In a few countries, citizens not of the "state religion" are persecuted, but in most countries there now exists religious freedom. It is more convenient to choose the "state religion"—the churches are more likely to be nearby, fewer questions are asked about "why" one believes, government and religious holidays match, products that support one's faith are more readily available in the stores. Yet, if one believes strongly in another faith, there is respect and encouragement.

When guiding a universal-computing environment, the "state religion" metaphor applies nicely. Communication is facilitated by standard computers using standard software and standard courseware. Yet, specific users (for example, graphic artists) may have special reasons not to adopt the standard, at least not for all they do. These outliers should be viewed with respect as they exercise with some inconvenience the strength of their preferences. It is important for an institution to declare the "state religion" in computers, for they are great advantages to standardization which can be more than 90 percent achieved on a voluntary basis if only the standard is known and conveniently accessible. At the same time, it is important that strongly convicted variation be accommodated.

• Teenagers Learning How to Drive

Learning new tricks is often all-consuming. When first learning how to drive a car, teenagers seem obsessed. They can quickly identify every car on the road. Talk about horsepower and engines and fuel alternatives is pervasive. Eventually, as the years pass, driving becomes routine. They no longer have to test the limits of their mechanical transporters. Concern can focus on "where they're going" instead of "the vehicle that is transporting them."

With computers in teaching and research, college faculties today manifest behaviors not unlike the teenagers. Suddenly, there is a powerful new tool for teaching, learning, and research. Its limits are unexplored. Its usage requires learning. And much of the talk in the halls and at conferences is not about the subject matter of their disciplines but instead about computers. As a profession, we are collectively (all ages) going through computer adolescence.

Soon the transition will end, and we can return to a focus on substance. Process will become routine. I can think about economics, not so much groupware techniques. In order to speed this desired transition, it behooves each of us to facilitate faculty learning about computers and to remind each other that this is indeed a stage which too will pass.

CHAPTER 4

THE BIG ISSUES

*"Pursue specific objectives within the
constraints of affordability."*

Resolving to implement "universal computing" accessible to all members of the community is an important first step. Between the dream and its realization, however, are many critical factors, or "big issues," that must be considered. Decisions must be made. The ultimate resolution of each of these issues rests primarily upon two premises: purpose and money.

An important first question to ask is "what are the primary purposes of providing universal computing throughout our community?" So many degrees of freedom exist! Yet, money spent increasing the capacity of the computer to support fancy lecture presentations cannot be also spent on more software applications, etc. To make wise choices between massive alternatives requires a clear understanding of the reasons university computing is being supplied to all community members.

"How much annually can the community afford to spend on the computing system?" Start up expenses include wiring, network servers, space renovations, training, programming systems, and updating individual work stations. Refreshing obsolete equipment, staffing support, reprogramming, printing are a beginning list of continuing expenses. Since the computer system is as strong as its weakest link; anticipation and planning are import to avoid overspending on the early elements. It is best to start with a ballpark figure and work within it. Once these limits are established, meaningful answers can be given to the why, what, and how issues.

WHY? ASSESSING GOALS AND NEEDS

What is it that you are trying to achieve? What strengths of your organization do you want to maximize? Upon what criteria should alternative configurations of computers be made?

• Identifying Your Primary Goals

If the primary goal is to facilitate communication, then standardizing systems (hardware, software, courseware), assuring a robust e-mail system, and providing a robust and flexible groupware program are important. If the primary objective is individualized Internet access, standardization becomes less crucial and there is an increased need for high-band width reaching the community. An emphasis upon analysis, such as statistical packages and spreadsheets, sometimes requires very heavy calculating capacity and rarely involves a need for standardization. An emphasis upon presentation suggests less investment in individual machines and more investment in projection, in Internet connectivity only for the presenter, in graphics capacities.

The recurring theme of this book is that the computer makes the greatest difference in the quality of life and the effectiveness of a community when it is viewed primarily as a communication device. Each community must, however, make its own decision and follow that decision with appropriate choices.

• Academic vs. Administrative

In most environments computers are used both to support the learning and research process (e.g., by faculty in courses) and to support administrative services (e.g., registering students and issuing payroll checks). In colleges we talk about "academic" and "administrative" computing. Often the two systems require very different capacities. Administrative systems, for example, usually require tighter security and involve tasks that are more likely to be repeated again and again, such as registration, newsletters, billing and paying, accounting, and word processing.

Since administrative uses are likely to be very structured and specific, whereas academic uses are likely to be much more diverse, as a general rule often broken, it may be best first to develop the academic uses of the computer, and then to adapt the system for business purposes. It is easier to narrow and focus the scope of an academic system than to broaden an administrative approach once it has been adopted.

• Virtual Medium vs. Mixed Media

What defines your community? Will some members be geographically remote, or unavailable at convenient times for the rest of the group? Will computer-based community supplement face-to-face communication, or will almost all communication be virtual?

Until new communication media have been tested by several generations of users, it is likely that the leaders of most communities will use the computer as one of several means of communication, not the sole means of communication. As more and more is learned about virtual communications, as better and better materials are developed, we can expect a migration toward distance learning, voting remotely, and sole reliance upon electronic databases. Until that time, most community developers will need to recognize the need for sustaining some of the traditional means of communicating, storing, and presenting information.

• Community Access and Information Flow

Are you seeking to maximize access by your community members to outside resources (the idea of a world of books available to all)? To maximize access by outsiders to your own community (e-commerce uses)? To enrich the communication solely within your community (access to a common database by a clearly defined group of users)?

Most communities require a spectrum of accesses. Some information will need to be available only to its author. Other information will need to be accessible to a clearly defined and restricted group of users (e.g., payroll information or student term papers). And there will be other times when issues of security, confidentiality, and even accuracy are less important. In general, communities defined for procedural purposes need to endure the inconvenience of restricted access, whereas communities defined for substantive purposes need to be more open, more accessible.

WHAT? STANDARDIZATION QUESTIONS

• Public vs. Network vs. Laptop vs. Desktop Computers

Your community's assumptions about the type of access that must be available to all members, as well as the type of use, will determine the ideal computer system. How much computing power will you need? How conveniently accessible must it be? How affordable?

For most communities (not taking account of cost), the ideal computer is very powerful, totally reliable, and available to everyone in the community at all times, even when travelling outside the normal bounds of the community. In a college community, this can mean very powerful, standardized laptop computers that are refreshed annually by top-rated vendors. Students, the privileged nomads of our society, can carry their computers off campus to internships, abroad, home during vacation, and off with them upon graduation.

Since most communities cannot afford the top of the line in all areas, nor do they need to rely upon all features equally, compromises deserve serious consideration. Since desktop computers are generally less expensive, is portability essential? (Are most members of the community "in place" or nomadic?) Since some brands are cheaper than others, how important is reliability and dependability (Can downtime be tolerated?)? Since "network computers" (i.e. vest pocket computers that can pick up e-mail and reach the Internet but have almost no calculating or storage capacity) are now available for under $500 and are much more convenient to carry around, does "connectivity" meet most of the community system demand? If "public computers" were located throughout the community like public telephones and the cost of individual ownership could be avoided, would 24-hour public access be an acceptable standard?

• Standard Hardware and Software vs. Freedom of Choice

The case for standardization of computers (all group members have the same, or one, of say, three computers) is very strong. One of the main advantages is mutual support. Students can learn from roommates, workers can learn from officemates, neighbors can share their knowledge. Orientation and special classes can be more sharply focused and taught by more knowledgeable individuals. Help desk and maintenance staff spend less time analyzing problems and implementing solutions. They can be trained in greater depth.

Another advantage is reliability. An errant machine can be quickly replaced from the loaner pool. Roommates can "look on" and even borrow computers when one of theirs is not working. By maintaining back-up computers at crucial locations (such as a classroom building), nearly instant substitution can be achieved. In those settings where all computers in the class must always be up and operating, reliability is an essential element in encouraging leaders to use the advantages of computer-enhanced communication.

Still another advantage is attitude. Professors can more confidently assume that all members of a class have access to a given level of computer capability and elevate their teaching standards and expectations accordingly. And students are much less likely to blame their inability to complete a task on the inadequacy of their computer and therefore much more likely to persevere.

On the other hand, standardization can be costly when one already has access to a computer (e.g., at work), when one doesn't need even the average level of computer power, when one switches from one community to another (e.g., high school to college), and where there are developmental advantages to being exposed to the "real world" of extremely diverse computers.

• Full Standardization vs. a Threshold Standard

Under what premise should the community operate? Should it pursue the threshold strategy by assuming that every member has 24-hour access to any computer (i.e., any brand, any power) that can operate a small number of specified programs (e.g., reach the internet by the current version of Netscape)? Or, are the training and reliability and maintenance advantages of a standard computer with standard software sufficient to justify the loss of flexibility and "individual discretion"?

Just as most community services are provided under the assumption that minimum transportation is available to all citizens, and most college courses are taught under the assumption that all students have access to the course's textbook; it is important for faculty to know what they may minimally expect of all students. By raising the expected threshold of computer access, the outcomes possible are also raised. A well-defined and fully articulated threshold standard is important.

- **Standard Courseware System or Course Shell**

Should standardization extend to the ways data is arranged? To the format for threaded discussions?

Many universities have adopted a "default" format for courses on the Web. They identify a common template (or set of templates) that can be modified to match the requirements of each course. At first most computer-intensive universities developed their own templates. Recently, due to the appearance of commercial packages such as Learning Space, WebCT, Web-Course-In-A-Box, Blackboard, and FrontPage, many of these same universities are migrating toward one of the commercial alternatives.

The concept of default formats is generally sound. Community members who learn how to navigate in one course (or committee or club or agency) can transfer that skill to another course that is using the same format. Students then spend less time learning "how to use the computer in a particular class" and more time on the subject matter of the class. Professors and other group leaders can avoid devoting one or two class periods to instructions about how to use the computer in this particular course. Members will be more proficient in their use of the computer.

The best "course shells" are extremely flexible. They provide a spectrum of "filing drawers" that differ by who has access to each drawer and what a person can do (submit, edit, delete) to documents in that drawer. Each system should support threaded discussions, provide a drawer that is accessible only to the author of the document (e.g. a professor's grade book drawer), and allow sub-groups to communicate privately with each other.

In most settings, acceptance of such default systems will depend on allowing computer experts and others with special needs to deviate from the standard format.

- **Mandatory vs. Optional**

Should owning the "right" computer be a mandatory condition for joining, or remaining part of, the group? In an environment committed to universal computing, it is essential that all members of the community act on the assumption that everyone has easy and unfettered access to an appropriate computer. Individuals joining these communities should be fully informed prior to joining, and once members, all should be subjected to the same mandatory requirement. In colleges, this same principle applies to textbooks.

The gains from standardizing equipment, software, groupware, and e-mail systems are immense. These gains occur in vendor leverage regarding price and preferred availability, in avoiding redundancy of training, in training knowledgeable help desk personnel, and in distributing and maintaining equipment. If at all possible, the basic student machine and its load should be standardized. Most faculty, as a matter of convenience and ease of communication with their students, will voluntarily conform to the student standard.

• Two Layers of Communication Utility

Many faculty and students will need access to two or more computers. The universal computer (for example, standard laptops) functions as the primary layer of computer access by facilitating communication and connectedness throughout the community. It will meet 99 percent of the other needs for computing as well. However, there will always be special-purpose needs that are beyond the capacity of "layer one" communication computers. Some of the "layer two" computers will contain data from old research projects. More often, they will be clustered in special laboratories where tasks like advanced computer imaging or enormous number-crunching tasks will be most efficiently pursued. The designation of a universal computer greatly reduces the need for general computer laboratories, but there will remain a need for specialized computers for special purposes. It is neither economical nor wise to expect the universal computer to be capable of completing every conceivable task.

How? Strategies for Implementation

• Consortia, Outsourcing, and Partnerships

Where are the economies in computing? Do consortia make sense? Where and how often should one outsource? Recognizing that a single university implements a major strategic plan for technology only about once a decade, and that the local experience base to solve largely new problems is limited, it behooves a university (or a community) to structure a pilot initiative that a vendor or group of vendors has a strong self-interest in seeing to success, or for a university to join up with kindred organizations (either other universities or geographically proximate institutions) to share expertise.

Outsourcing is routine. Candidates for project outsourcing include writing code for specialized programs, designing Web pages, routine training, and highly sophisticated decisions about system design. Typically not outsourced are program development (i.e. assistance in designing specific applications), server space, and faculty-staff development. Few institutions can afford full time access to the full spectrum of specialized computer expertise.

Consortia make the most sense where a bond among institutions already exists. At the moment, technology enabled cost-effective small servers and the economies of scale in the equipment domain are few. Increasingly, however, there are likely to be consortia of help desks and similar functions.

• General Contractor (Single Vendor) vs. Multiple Contractors

What are the advantages and disadvantages of long term relationships with a single vendor or cluster of vendors? Does our community wish to identify a single vendor's machine as preferred?

Here the forces of politics and economics converge. Several advantages accrue from a long-term contract with a trusted vendor, most likely the producer of the student computer. Among these advantages are early alerts concerning upcoming products, favored availability and reliability of delivery, decreased likelihood of incompatibilities among components of the system, and access to consulting resources when challenges outdistance local expertise.

Computer systems are complex. From the perspective of the university or college, it is best for a vendor with broad experience in such systems to have a stake in the success of a local system. Often these primary vendors can exert some leverage upon other vendors and subcontractors. Usually they can help locate specialized expertise to join in a consulting effort.

However, especially in public institutions, it is often impolitic to select a single vendor. In some instances, where the number of computers to be purchased is very large, there may also be some bargaining price advantage to using more than one vendor.

• Top Down vs. Participatory Approval: Centralized Support vs. Decentralized

What is the successful strategy for implementing universal computing? Once the decision is made to go universal, are the support mechanisms best centralized or decentralized?

In colleges and universities most of the early adoptions of universal computing are in settings where the president, or another authority, has inherited or earned substantial authority and is able to lead the community without passing through the votes of numerous panels and committees. The commitment to universal computing is so costly and often so disruptive that it cannot be implemented without strong support and leadership from the top.

Yet, leaders of each sub-community need to feel a sense of ownership in the decision to adopt universal computing. In a university, the decision is best processed through the faculty governance system, for it is individual professors who lead each classroom "community." If, on the other hand, the universal system is to be used primarily for business functions (e.g. registration, invoicing), top-down approval makes the most sense. It depends.

Experienced administrators of universal computing systems are nearly unanimous in their belief that a support system cannot be either exclusively centralized or exclusively decentralized. In a university, for example, requests for help can be made to a central help desk, and questions not answered there can be referred back to the department for more intense consideration. With equal success, the department may be the point of first inquiry, with a centralized follow-up at a central help desk for specialized questions. Because there are needs both for quick answers to simple questions and thoughtful answers to more difficult questions, a mixed approach is best.

• **Phased & Piloted Implementation**

Is it possible and/or wise to implement "universal computing" for a portion of a community? How essential is it to develop experience through a pilot program before adopting a full-scale community model?

A significant portion of the benefits from universal computing cannot be realized until all members are part of the system. The incentive for simultaneous adoption is high and the rewards can be great. Usually, however, the "all at once" strategy backfires because small organizations cannot mount, construct and maintain a complex implementation without experiencing major glitches. Unless the community is small, homogeneous, and forgiving, a phased implementation is recommended.

The phasing can be by sector (government social service agencies or the business school within a university), by geography (neighborhood or building), or by cohort (fifth grade or freshmen first). By limiting scale and impact, it is often possible to work through the would-be glitches before they become major crises. Phasing also allows organizations to alert newcomers to the higher fees needed to support many computer initiatives, while leaving continuing participants at their familiar fee schedule. On college campuses, several student-protests against higher fees have been averted by such a strategy.

• **Start with Budget Boundary**

Only a few universities have had any success adjusting their budgets to accommodate a universal computing activity that is headed toward taking roughly 6 percent of an institution's budget. This is a new expenditure, one that is too large to be easily accommodated within existing budgets.

All universities have constraints. Just as it makes no sense to design a new academic building for which there is absolutely no prospect of funding, it is equally unwise to design computer systems that can't be funded. The best way to proceed is to identify up front the maximum amount that might become available for computing, and then to write a 5 to 10 year plan that fits within that budget.

Keep in mind that until recently, computer equipment was treated as long-term capital. With the realization that computers become obsolete in two years, computer expenditures must increasingly be viewed as recurrent and annual. They should, therefore be written into operating, not capital, budgets.

• **Ignore Sunk Costs**

In recent years the rate of computer obsolescence has been more rapid than automobiles and clothing. Over two years, today's laptops lose about 75 percent of their initial value. Older computers often can't handle newly authored software. We enter an economist's dream world where only marginal or new costs and marginal or new benefits are relevant. At first, Wake Forest struggled to get its 486 processors back into the central warehouse, only to find that no one else wanted the now-obsolete machines. When making decisions about computing, it is best to ignore "sunk costs" and choose alternatives that make the most sense for the future.

• **Buy Computers vs. Lease vs. Students Buy**

Should the town, the school, or the college buy computers and assign them to students? Should it arrange for the computers to be leased directly by the vendor to the group members? Should it encourage group members to buy on their own?

All arrangements seem to work, especially if the specifications are rigorous and specific. The decision often rests on the terms of the contract between the vendor and the institution, and on the availability of capital to the college or school system or community.

Putting it All Together

The ultimate communication system evolves when all community members have 24-hour, 7-day-a-week access to the Internet. At this time over 50 colleges and universities have pursued such a strategy. Ray Brown, Executive Director of the Associated Colleges of Central Kansas, maintains a list of these diverse institutions at http://www.acck.edu/ray/NoteBookList.htm.

Each of these institutions has crafted its own strategy. Each institution has resolved "the big issues" to match its mission, constituency, and circumstance. As an illustration, the chart below summarizes the principles that most shaped the decisions at Wake Forest.

DECISION CONCEPTS AT WAKE FOREST	
Students First	Marketable Difference
Communication Emphasis	Eager Faculty
Academic Before Administrative	Exposure not Mandate
Breadth of Usage Before Depth	Multiple Units Win
Standard Student Computers	Starting Budget Limit
Standard Student Load	Operating Budget
Dominant Use After Graduation	Sunk Cost Ignored
Students as Nomads	Partnership
Academic Freedom	Rapid Change
Students as Change Agents	Two Layers of Computers

Much emphasis has been placed upon focussed decision making. When establishing computer strategies, literally thousands of micro-decisions influence the character of the system. For example, on which software systems can one cut corners and where is it wise to invest in the best? What's the best strategy for printing? Is round-the-clock staffing of the help desk essential? Thousands of decisions are to be made, by dozens of people, and the choices will either reinforce or frustrate the central intentions for the system.

Leadership's responsibility is to define and communicate a finite set of basic concepts against which each micro-decision can be tested. These concepts will differ greatly from one college/community to another. These concepts are necessary quite "individualized" to each situation.

Chapter 5

Achieving a Reasonable Consensus

"The procedural fundamentals for achieving faculty approval for change in academic policy must be honored."

The strategic cycle for the consideration and implementation of a technology initiative is long and complex. It may be helpful to think of the cycle as having four phases: decision, implementation, adoption, and evaluation.

During the decision phase, both an institutional aspiration and its opportunities inform broad strategic choices. Sub-phases might include identification of the issue and definition of the questions, conceptualization of broad alternatives, advancement of a primary strategy, and discussion and buy-in by major stakeholders. During the implementation phase, sub-phases might include preparation of infrastructure, especially personnel and networks and choice, distribution, and maintenance of student access computers. During the adoption phase, sub-phases might include basic training for students and faculty users of computers, and exposure, exploration, experimentation and adoption by faculty. During the evaluation phase, sub-phases might include collection and analysis of assessment data, and revision and revisitation of the decision phase.

In this and the next two chapters, our focus shifts from the most important decisions of what and why to the time-consuming tasks of consensus building and course design.

Fundamental Rules

There is no magic bullet. Gaining consensus from multiple stakeholders on the allocation of vast sums of new money will always be a challenge. However, strategies based upon the two following rules are more likely to succeed:

• The Decision to Adopt Universal Computing Needs to be Treated as an Academic Rather Than a Financial or Administrative One

The mere extension of administrative systems to include course databases doesn't work, neither technically nor psychologically.

Faculty rightfully need to feel in control of all aspects of their teaching environment.

• Technology is No Exception: The Procedural Fundamentals for Achieving Faculty Approval for Change in Academic Policy Must be Honored.

In the minds of faculty, and in reality, computers are a major factor in shaping academic achievement. The computer infrastructure, much like the library, is a basic educational resource. The same faculties claiming jurisdiction over matters such as grading policy, curriculum content, and library purchasing strategies will expect similar faculty authority to be exercised in the computer domain, at least as they relate to computers used in the classroom and in research.

TECHNIQUES FOR BUILDING CONSENSUS

From these two fundamental rules grow a set of suggestions that follows:

• Follow Established Routes Of Approval

At a Midwestern medical school that provided laptop computers to all students five years ago, these computers have yet to be used significantly in the classroom. The finance division thought that computers were important and, without consultation or discussion, found a way to pay for them. Here, the problem was that faculty and students not only didn't have an opportunity to shape the decision, they felt an invasion into territory previously "owned" by academics. By open discussions and normal voting in standing committee, such resistances can be avoided.

• Keep Everyone Informed

Most of all, in colleges and universities this refers to faculty. Students, alumni, governing board members, and legislatures and donors all expect to know what is happening in this rapidly developing domain. Computers themselves, through e-mail, open new possibilities not only for spreading rumors but also for countering them. Periodic updates (perhaps every two weeks during active consideration) of a brief newsletter from the Dean (or another respected academic) go a long way in establishing trust. Use the technology!

• Allow Ample Time and Request Feedback, to the Point of Redundancy

Faculties relish disclosure and full discussion, especially when there is a valid sense that good new ideas will be reflected in final outcomes. Everyone must believe they have been given an opportunity to comment on the intended course of action. In academe, the opportunity to comment is a "birthright." Most won't comment and, as a consequence of having had the opportunity, will join the consensus. In recent years, many colleges have issued rough drafts of strategic planning reports on newsprint in order to emphasize the roughness of the draft, held hearings and invited feedback via other formats; eventually, after everyone has had their say, they have issued a revised final report.

• Use the Peer Culture

When making complex judgments, many of us find it easier to rely upon a trusted representative than to reach an independent decision. The best way to "sell" a technology plan is to recruit trusted peers (disciplinary peers, age-cohort peers, neighborhood peers, value-based peers, etc.) to talk among themselves. The Wake Forest Technology Plan would never have been adopted were it not for an originally very skeptical group of computer-knowledgeable faculty who eventually became the primary advocates of the plan.

• Recognize Diversity

Disciplines and subcommunities use computers in vastly different ways. Scientists need number-crunching machines that can, among other things, monitor experiments. Social scientists most often use the spreadsheet and the communicating capacities of computers. Humanists often seek access to obscure (to America) foreign-language texts, need sorting strategies for vast databases accumulated over centuries, and encourage students to study abroad. The arts require massive computer capacities to handle video and sound. Medical and legal educators express special concern for confidentiality and privacy. Taken together, the disciplines have very different needs, all of which need to be accounted for when designing both a computer strategy and a strategy for the approval of a plan.

• **Empower Many Agencies Throughout the Organization**

Faculties become understandably anxious about potential shifts in "power and influence," both within the faculty and beyond it. Most technology plans specify additional hires, and budget augmentations. By, for example, asking the library to take responsibility for basic computer training of students and faculty, asking the bookstore to distribute new computers, providing each department with a new computer technician, centering budget dollars for new disciplinary software at the dean's or department chair's office, establishing an elected committee to set computer policy, authorizing additional residence-hall staff to advise students on computer usage, and charging the IS department itself with implementation responsibility for only a portion of the new plan; much of the anxiety about one unit becoming too large and powerful can be averted. Moreover, if the support units stand to gain staff positions if the technology plan is approved, they may well become advocates among peer units.

• **Honor Heritage**

The benefits of standardization (i.e. adopting a single computer system) often outweigh the costs. Even so, it is wise to tolerate some lingering diversity. Many faculty, for example, have their research data on a "legacy" system and do not have the time or expertise to transfer the data to a new system. In addition, learning a new system takes time that may not be available in any given month. Approval strategies must include assurances that legacy systems will be supported before being phased out and that phase-out periods will be realistically flexible. Allowing current faculty and staff to "control" the disposition of their outdated computers can be an inexpensive (the old computer isn't worth much anyway) and effective means of gaining support for a new initiative.

• **Consider a "Package" of Changes**

In most representative bodies significant legislation emerges from compromise and trade-off. Party A will honor Party B's passion if, especially if in the same bill, Party B honors Party A's passion. At this point in time, different stakeholders and sub-stakeholder constituencies place very different values upon technological restructuring. Science faculty, trustees, and students by and large place a greater value upon new computers and networks. Other stakeholders see more value in allocating resources to hire more faculty, in offering better student scholarships, in subscribing to more publications or buying more research equipment. By fashioning five-to-ten-year academic plans, not unlike then-year capital campaigns, it is often possible to accommodate several passions. By linking funding commitments to multifaceted strategic plans that include a technology upgrade as one item in the package, more passions can be accommodated. Approval of an entire plan becomes more probable.

- **Visit Other Campuses**

From group visits to other campuses, members of a faculty-administrative committee like deTocqueville can gain perspective on the "home" culture. They invariably spot good ideas and develop common vocabularies. Most of all, the fellow travelers come to know each other better. They come to know what is most important to each other. Benefiting from the catalytic effect of seeing another system, they are to reflect upon the whole range of issues associated with an ambitious technology initiative.

- **Be Lucky**

Lucky timing is crucial. The wrong newspaper headlines immediately prior to a crucial vote can kill an initiative. A new product announcement made only days after commitments have been made to what is now destined to be obsolete before it reaches campus. Extraordinary unhappiness over an unrelated issue by one of the stakeholder constituencies. The death or resignation of a champion for a particular plan or of a key representative in the vendor community. All of these things and more can go wrong. But conversely, events like the chairman of the board's implementing a computer plan in her company, a feature on a faculty champion who is using computers successfully in her class, the adoption of a technology plan by a nearby college or community can operate in favor of adoption. One must recognize that windows of opportunity stay open only so long, and that when they are important it is important to lead deliberation toward a timely conclusion.

CONCLUSION

Shepherding strategic technology plans through colleges and communities is successful when the basic procedures and mores of the community are understood and honored. Without a basic foundation of trust, change cannot occur. Involving whole communities in major decisions is time consuming but essential.

Chapter 6

Faculty Development Strategies for Encouraging the Actual Use of Computers in Teaching

". . . faculty are eager to consider the use of technology to enhance their instructional effectiveness."

In the last thirty years there has never been a time when so many faculty, and so many disciplinary professional associations, have been thinking so much about teaching — what's taught, what should be taught, and how it is best taught. The value systems of the profession have swung toward rewarding effort and success in teaching.

The new emphasis upon teaching should not be a surprise. Of foremost concern to faculty has always been how students learn. Virtually all members of our profession are open to new ideas and are quick to consider the usefulness of new methodologies as soon as they appear. The apparent indifference to teaching that over-shadowed the profession for the past fifty years has been more the result of "more of the same old" and of the absence of any major innovation opportunities.

With computerization has come the opportunity to use very different teaching methods. Degrees of freedom have been radically expanded. In such an environment it makes sense that faculty would take the time to rethink what they are doing and why, to consider all ways they might improve (including non-technological ways), and then to fashion new strategies that mix in what they find to be the most successful new tools.

Faculty development programs should be based on the assumption that faculties will be pushing IS departments to support course redesign, and that IS departments face the challenge not to motivate faculty, but rather to keep up with faculty who are already being motivated by their peers and their profession.

It is neither necessary nor wise to mandate the adoption in all disciplines by all professors for all students the use of still yet barely tested techniques. The mores of the professions will push adoption forward as fast as is desirable.

Changing teaching habits is time-intensive, risky, and difficult. Even so, many faculty throughout the country are quickly and courageously experimenting with computer-enhanced instruction. Many of these experiments are being vigorously supported by well-reasoned, imaginative faculty development programs. This chapter focuses upon these programs.

THE CHARACTER OF FACULTY CULTURE

Although each campus has its own ethos and each leader has his or her own style, there are several universal traits that define "faculty culture." Understanding these traits can meaningful shape strategies for exposing more faculty to ways that computers can be used to increase their instructional effectiveness.

• Environmental Imperatives

Before faculty members can "afford" wide-scale experimentation with computer-based learning, they must "believe in" the reliability and equity of the system. They must believe that their students will not be disadvantaged by their experiments.

Pragmatically this means that (1) the computers and their networks must run reliably, (2) all students in the class must have universal and nearly equal access to computers, (3) multiple opportunities for training and help-desk consultation must be convenient and inexpensive, and (4) a faculty ethos must exist that values experimentation and tolerates missteps. Without these basic assurances, faculty will not undertake the difficult task of reworking their heretofore successful teaching strategies.

Fairness and equity require that all students have equal access to essential learning tools such as textbooks, the library, and computers. Redundancies must be built into systems of access to assure computer availability when equipment breaks or batteries become dead. Professors will avoid technology when too many of their students fail to complete homework assignments because the technology is broken.

Reliable networks are equally important. Professors and students will stop sending e-mail messages if the delivery system lacks predictability. Professors will appropriately step back from the use of technology if the network is down during class. Even two lost minutes at the front of a classroom populated by forty students feels like an eternity. If networks are so unreliable that alternative plans must be made for each class session, there is significant disincentive for experimentation and adoption.

Universal access to equipment and training and consultation, predictable and reliable networks for communication, and a vibrant culture that encourages experimentation are prerequisites for a successful usage strategy.

Over centuries a primary contribution of universities has been their capacity to house simultaneously persons of diametrically opposing views. Universal computing must be implemented in ways that do not endanger this essential dimension of all good universities and colleges. Specifically, the activities of research laboratories and classrooms should be "off limits" to browsing stakeholders. The developmental essays written by students in their early years often need to be perishable, in ways that the ideas that are testing do not become a permanent part of their profile and digital persona. Encryption and password-protected accesses are important.

• Eager Faculty

The vast majority of faculty are eager to consider the use of technology to enhance their instructional effectiveness. The availability of these new methods has sparked a national conversation about teaching methods, a conversation that is driving what may be the most thorough self-examination of teaching and learning experienced in the 20th century. Faculty culture is applauding the conscientious consideration and adoption of technology. Finding extra time to learn new methods is a problem; motivating the desire to explore is not. .

It is neither necessary nor wise to mandate the adoption in all disciplines by all professors for all students the use of still yet barely tested techniques. The mores of the professions will push adoption forward as fast as is desirable.

• Faculty Ownership

The adoption of computers will spread by "word of mouth" among faculty. Initially it is important for the faculty of a college, and of a discipline, to mutually agree that the dollar and time investment in technology is a worthy risk (for example, by an all-faculty vote). Primary encouragement for testing the use of technology must be faculty-to-faculty, with administrators sitting on the sidelines. Building and maintaining channels of communication, both within a faculty and among faculties, is crucial. Information about computer-enhanced learning is most trusted when it comes from traditional sources such as teaching colleagues, disciplinary associations and meetings, and library professionals.

- **Centrality of Educational Theory**

    Educational theory must drive the adoption of technology, not vice versa. When redesigning courses, the instructor-innovator must first identify beliefs about how students learn best, how the particularity of the material is best conveyed, and what the most essential role of the instructor is. Then, and only then, is it possible to consider what approaches, newly enabled by technology, should be pursued. For example, how can the computer be used to increase the level of trust between mentor and learner? In what ways can the computer facilitate collaboration among learners? How important is access to original source materials and, if deemed important, how can such access be facilitated by computers? Is immediate feedback important and, if so, how can the computer facilitate it? To what extent should students structure their own learning experiences? How important is frequent exchange between students and faculty and among students?

- **Communication**

    Education is fundamentally communication between learner and mentor. The mentor may be the instructor, a student colleague, a knowledgeable alum assisting with the course, an expert on another continent, or an author from another era. The power of the computer is similar to the power of the telephone: it facilitates communication. Because communication can be asynchronous as well as synchronous, because messages may be videos and sounds as well as words and symbols; the computer is the grand new communication facilitator. It is the power to enhance communication, not fancy classroom presentations or even faster analyses, that is driving the paradigm shift that the computer represents.

• **Hybrid Instruction**

The widespread adoption of computers in learning will first occur as a component of traditional courses taught to schoolchildren and college students in residence. Treated as resources like libraries and laboratories, computers will be used when appropriate and not used when not appropriate. The most readily accepted use of computers will be as enhancements of traditional behaviors, such as the use of e-mail to communicate more frequently and sometimes more substantively with more students. Within a few years most resident college students will use computers much as they use textbooks today, as fully integrated into virtually all of their courses. Within a typical course, some material will best be presented by the computer and some by the class leader, in person. Although computers are becoming an increasingly important component in distance learning, they will not become fully accepted until tested and proven in residential environments.

• **Friends Teach Each Other**

Like speaking a language and driving a car, instruction in "how to operate a computer" is helpful. Most learning, however, occurs by observing others, by coaching from friends, or by getting answers on a "need to know" basis. Many students come from high school willing to share their computer knowledge with their friends and professors. When all students "speak the same language" or use the same computers, friends help friends learn. Officemates share. Roommates share. Classmates share. Such sharing is greatly facilitated by compatible, ideally standardized equipment and software. By establishing modal standards for the ways in which computers are used, learning through sharing is increased and at the same time (since learning new computer skills is not required with each new class) the total amount of learning that must occur is reduced.

• **Flexibility**

There is no "cookie-cutter" pattern for a single methodology of best teaching. Requirements vary by discipline, by subject matter, by professor, by student, or by circumstance. Some work is best done in student teams, some not. Some lectures are best studied in advance of the class, some not. Some graded essays are best shared with the whole class, some not. Some classes are enhanced by viewing the work by students enrolled in previous semesters, some not. Each instructor teaches in different ways. Guidelines for the standardized use of computers must facilitate this diversity.

Scholars and creative talents greatly value their capacity to reach original sources and to understand procedures influencing outcomes. Guidelines for standardization must allow faculty to "do it their way" without massive commitments of personal time. Standardized training formats that can be altered only by dedicated computer professionals will not gain acceptance among faculty who are accustomed to far more flexibility and control.

• Diversity among Disciplines

The "computer explosion" will proceed at different rates in different domains of knowledge, based upon factors such as copyrights, the character of information, the geographic proximity of subspecialists, and the skill sets emphasized by each discipline. New teaching methods will be adopted most rapidly if faculty lead at rates appropriate for their individual disciplines and subspecialities.

• Innovation is Threatening

Important avant-garde and unfamiliar uses of technology for learning enhancement should first be tested and showcased in a unit not responsible for the overall success of ongoing programs. Research and development in experimental classes involves risks to the students that are unacceptably high to most professors. New methods should first be tested among smaller sets of consenting learners.

• Patience

It is tempting for faculty innovators and administrators to measure the percentage of faculty "adopting" these powerful new methods, and to view non-adoption as failure. Far more constructive is the realization that all innovations need time to mature, that reticence among some faculty is wisdom, and that truly successful enhancements will soon become nearly universally adopted. The strategic campaign should be directed toward exposure and consideration of technology; not measured in any one year against an "adoption" rate.

It is unimportant and perhaps undesirable that every faculty member utilize this technology. It is essential, however, that every faculty member understand the opportunities provided by the computer, have support in designing and experimenting with computer enhancements to their instruction, and make informed choices based on the availability of the full range of instructional methodologies.

STRATEGIES THAT ENCOURAGE EXPLORATION AND USE

Once computers are used at home or at the office, their use for instruction flows naturally. Communities should build systems that reinforce computer usage by enabling the skills developed for one purpose to migrate easily to other purposes. Ways to encourage reinforcing computer use are listed below.

• **E-mail**

Increasingly communication among subspecialists throughout the world is backboned by e-mail. An easy-to-use, totally reliable, fully accessible, full-featured e-mail system will lure even the most reluctant to turn on and start using their computers. Soon e-mail messages will be flowing between professors and their students.

• **Use Outside the Classroom**

As a means of encouraging all who wish to participate to learn computing fundamentals, departmental minutes and faculty committee documents can be generated electronically By encouraging the playful exploration of the World Wide Web, the use of computers by members of student organizations and athletic teams and the organization of research materials in electronic files, a campus can advance computer skill level and therefore facilitate instructional use.

• **Policy of Universal Access.**

Each instructor needs to know the threshold level of computing that may be expected of each student. Is it fair to assume that every student has a very powerful computer and knowledge adequate to access a live network at all times, and that he or she will be connected to the network during class? If not, what can be expected? Until an instructor can reliably assume a reasonable level of universal access, course redesign must be constrained to accommodate the computerless.

• Standardization of Equipment and Software

By standardizing software and hardware, faculty and students can help each other through equipment failures and learning challenges. Such reliability encourages use. Roommates teach each other. Faculty colleagues share more easily. Although standardization is difficult for all campuses to achieve, standardizing students' equipment (especially by providing leased computers) establishes a threshold upon which faculty and students can rely. Faculty are likely voluntarily to choose the student standard for themselves.

• Standard Filing System

Many campuses are encouraging all faculty to place course materials in electronic file cabinets which have a common structure. For example, each "file cabinet" may contain a "drawer" for the syllabus, another drawer for reserve reading materials, another drawer for threaded discussions, another drawer for the private storage of materials related to the course, and so on. By establishing this common standard, which is conveniently accessible, each professor can avoid teaching students how the computer is to be used in their individual class, and each student can quickly master access to the data related to the course. Instructors who believe they cannot afford to give up two lectures on Elizabethan literature in order to introduce computer usage for their particular course do not need to do so.

• The Basic Service Philosophy

If a community is to afford threshold computing for all its members, it may have to restrict unwarranted and casual overusage of the system by a few individuals. This can be achieved by establishing charges for extraordinarily heavy usage—for example, big printing jobs and heavily animated personal web pages.

• **Portability**

Most professors prepare for class in their office and teach their class in another location, the classroom. Most students go to class in a different location than where they study. Significant time is saved when the same computer can be carried to all locations. Reliability is also increased. More reliable computing in less time is a significant incentive for adoption.

• **Access from Home**

For most faculty and many students, considerable work is done at home or at off campus housing. If the computer is to be a universal tool, access to campus networks must be provided from these locations. At Wake Forest we pay the monthly fee for all faculty who wish to subscribe to an Internet provider such as IGN or AOL. Students may access our network from off campus through an often crowded modem pool or by paying for monthly access through our contract with IGN.

• **Academic Policy**

Technology presents new opportunities for plagiarism, for collaboration, and for very rapid communication. Individual faculty members should not have to deal with establishing new *ad hoc* policies simply because they are early adopters of the computer. A faculty committee, preferably elected, should articulate these policies for the community at large.

Taken together, these strategies emphasize four things: the importance of reliability, setting specific expectations for all members of the community, drawing people into using computers, and reducing the individual investment of time required to achieve adequate proficiency levels. The campus examples cited here apply equally to schools and towns.

A Key to Success: The "Low-Hanging Fruit"

To achieve necessary political and economic support for computer initiatives, the early involvement of a large percentage of the faculty is crucial. Faculty development programs can either emphasize helping the "eagles" (the early adopters of technology) to refine and extend their use of technology, or emphasize encouraging the "mid- to late-adopters" to incorporate into their teaching low effort, high return computer tools, the "low hanging fruit."

The highest returns come from tools that emphasize improved communication. At Wake Forest where computers are universal, over 80 percent of all students and faculty report that the quality and quantity of their interactions (students with faculty, students with other students, faculty with other faculty) has increased dramatically. The reported impact of PowerPoint presentations, of computer based exercises, and even of increased access to Internet data was, at best, half as large.

There are three easy-to-learn, computer-based teaching tools that can enrich communication. These are (1) group e-mail, (2) URLs or Internet addresses, and (3) electronic file cabinets (including the capacity for threaded conversations) for each course. By requiring that each student check e-mail each day and promising equal diligence from the instructor, communication about the subject matter of a particular course can be virtually continuous throughout a semester. By asking students to develop a list of Internet sites containing information relevant to a particular course, each student is provided access to alternative sources of information, often in more familiar (to them) multimedia format. Electronic file cabinets can place lecture notes, video clips, previous semesters' term papers, supplemental readings, reserve materials, profiles and photographs of class member, and grade term papers, all in one place where they can easily be found and conveniently kept for future reference.

These three tools in combination can be learned by an e-mail user in less than ninety minutes. After determining those aspects of teaching that should be enriched, it is most logical to ask first if there are ways that any or all of the "low hanging fruit" can be useful. There will be other uses of computers, such as providing access to materials on CD-ROM, but these three uses are likely to be the most universal and to quickly yield positive returns from the investment of time and money in computers.

WAYS TO ENCOURAGE INFORMATION EXCHANGE

According to Moore's Law, computing capacity doubles every eighteen months. In such a dynamic period extraordinary effort is required of faculty who must not only maintain the authenticity of teaching by established methods on tested and trusted information bases but also must explore and evaluate, even eventually learn, new data sources and new techniques. In a fast moving world, information exchange becomes even more important. The next ten strategies emphasize sharing.

- **Swap and Share Sessions**

    Every campus has its early adopters. Perhaps in a knowledge series of breakfast meetings or poster sessions or fortnightly afternoon seminars, the early adopters should share their experiences with colleagues throughout the campus.

- **Benchmarking Trips**

    Several times each year, a delegation of faculty should be encouraged to travel as a group to another campus, where they can observe and discuss with colleagues in their own discipline how technology is enhancing learning. Members of the visiting delegation can also spend a great deal of time talking with one another about computer enhancements.

- **On-Campus Workshops Led by Visiting Experts**

    Every month or so, an early adopter from another college or university should be invited to share ideas and experiences in an open seminar.

- **Best Practices Conference**

    A variant of the visiting speaker/consultant concept, three or four experts (usually from another campus) can be asked to talk about practices at their institution, and about future trends, while three or four local leaders eavesdrop. Invariably these conversations turn to how to identify the best practices for the local community and how to apply them.

- **Computer Tip Talk**

    Individual professors can ask their students to guide other students toward meaningful computer usage. For example, chemistry students can be asked to search for Web sites relevant to the course. In an economics class, each student can be asked to make a ten-minute presentation on a specific computer topic relevant to the course (for example, accessing the library catalogue, preparing a PowerPoint demonstration, downloading from the Web, or creating a Web page).

- **Subsidized Attendance at National Computer Meetings**

At most universities, travel funds are allocated by department chairs for participation in disciplinary meetings. For faculty to also attend meetings centered on computers and the use of instructional technologies, separate, new conference funding must be identified. At least in the initial years, these funds are probably best allocated from the dean's office for the explicit purpose of attendance at meetings where technology, not academic discipline, is the primary focus.

- **Training on Call**

New Wake Forest students receive their computers and a training disk at home before enrolling as freshmen. During orientation, three hours of computer training is required. Throughout the semester noncredit classes, usually lasting between one and three hours, are offered around the heavily used software programs (Microsoft Word, Lotus Notes, Excel, Netscape, etc.). Also we have online roughly two hundred self-guided training modules, each relating to a specific software usage. In spite of all these opportunities, most students and faculty seek training "just in time" and in response to a specific need. Because the ways in which students and faculty use computers are so diverse, common training strategies and times don't work very well. Much individual instruction is required. Training upon request, especially for a particular class, must be viewed as "ordinary and expected."

- **Summer Workshops**

Three-day summer workshops for faculty focus upon topics such as Using the Computer to Support Collaborative Learning, Setting Up a New Course on the Computer, Enhancing Writing Instruction Through the Computer, and Establishing a Web Page for Research and Teaching Purposes. The organizers of these workshops are faculty members. Workshop attendance is encouraged, when possible, by giving priority to workshop participants for securing a scheduled upgrade in their personal computers.

- **Electronic Resource File**

    When community members (for example, all faculty in an academic department) spot an article or a Web page that they feel would be of general interest, they should be able to place it in an electronic file cabinet that is accessible by all, and then inform others.

AGENCIES FOR ENCOURAGING COMPUTER ADOPTION

A motto might be "different strokes for different folks." A successful faculty development structure must be multifaceted. Computer advice must come from sources that are trusted, available at all hours, appropriately equipped, and knowledgeable. Different faculty groups will use different agencies. Each community must seek its own mix. Listed below are several types of agencies that have proven to be successful in their setting.

- **Academic Computer Specialists**

    Place in each academic building a disciplinary trained and computer knowledgeable individual who is responsible for assisting faculty and students in a discipline or cluster of disciplines. This person is hired by and reports to the department chairs. Typically the academic computer specialists are most intimately involved in the development of computer usages for specific courses.

- **Student Technology Assistants**

    Students should be given significant opportunities to assist faculty in course design, Web page development, and other projects. There are many models. The Student Technology Advisors' Program (STARS) at Wake Forest selects fifty freshmen or sophomore students and puts them through ten hours per week of paid training for an entire semester. The highly trained students are then individually assigned to a different professor each semester for the purpose of helping him or her enhance courses and their research through the adoption of the computer. These students are typically assigned to mid- and late-adopter faculty and are typically more knowledgeable then the faculty members. Special efforts are made to provide summer internships for these STARS, both as in-service training and as valuable entries on their postgraduation resumes. A second corps of twenty students serves as computer experts housed throughout the residence hall system. Their responsibility is to answer specific questions concerning computer usage addressed to them by students in their residence hall, questions that often come to them at unusual hours.

• Library Trainers

At Wake Forest, responsibility for computer classes is centered in the university library. Most classes are held in the library. Five staff members were added to the library for the explicit purpose of training, and a number of librarians, previously on the staff, have undergone extensive supplemental training so they too can conduct classes. When there is a need for concentrated training, such as during student orientation, and for specialized training, the librarians often involve the academic computer specialists.

• Computer Enhanced Learning Initiative

At most universities either an associate provost or a staff member within a Center for Teaching and Learning has primary responsibility for encouraging and facilitating the use of technology in teaching. An alternative approach, which has the twin advantages of "coming from within the faculty" and avoiding an entrenched point-of-view that emphasizes how the computer is used in a subset of disciplines, is the creation of an all-faculty committee. At Wake Forest the five faculty members of this committee, the Computer Enhanced Learning Initiative (CELI), serve for five semesters. Each semester a different member, freed from all teaching responsibilities, chairs the committee. The full committee meets regularly to create and implement particular programs that encourage faculty exploration of using computers for instruction. Each director focuses upon two or three specific programs, and all directors organize swap and share sessions and benchmarking trips. For example, the director for one semester, an assistant professor of mathematics and computer Science, focused on computer enhanced writing instruction, the use of threaded discussions, and the creation of electronic journals. The director for another semester focused on establishing Web pages for individuals and courses, on a common Web-based template for courses, and on multimedia uses of the computer. In still another semester, the focus will be on the creation of self-directed learning exercises in the sciences.

By passing around the leadership of CELI, each disciplinary user group is given its semester in the spotlight. Empowering former and future directors to work as a policy-setting team also assures continuity.

- **Committee on Information Technology**

It is important that users name a representative group that has the authority to recommend or make basic policy decisions. This elected faculty committee advises the administration regarding the features desired in the standard computer, the standard software load, and it sets faculty policy related to the computer.

- **Deans and Department Chairs**

Special funds should be established at the discretion of dean (or in larger institutions, department chair) for supporting equipment and software purchases. By including these allocations as a normal part of the budget process, the advantages of decentralized decision making can be realized.

- **Information Systems and the Help Desk**

Information systems should be responsible for establishing and maintaining the network and for staffing the "round-the-clock" information desk. Maintenance and distribution of computers is another responsibility of information systems. Spare computers should be housed in most academic buildings so that breakdowns in the midst of class sessions can be mitigated by loaner computers.

- **Instructional Laboratories**

Many campuses have created "outpatient clinics" where faculty can drop in to use sophisticated equipment (e.g., high quality scanners) and gain advice from well-trained experts. Such laboratories are especially important at those campuses where presentation and the original development of course materials are emphasized.

SUMMARY

To succeed, an initiative for faculty usage must be faculty led, student facilitated, multifaceted, and well supported.

CHAPTER 7

RELATING EDUCATIONAL THEORY AND TECHNOLOGY

"The important issue is how to improve
teaching and learning, not technology."

The sudden availability of many new computer-based teaching tools challenges each of us to rethink our teaching strategies. Each teacher, each learner, each community member must determine where, if anywhere, the technology can be used in ways to increase benefits more than costs. The important issue is how to improve teaching and learning, not how to justify dollars spent on technology. The sudden availability of many new computer-based learning tools is a strong reason to be rethinking teaching strategies at this time. The reconsideration may or may not result in the use of computers.

To rethink fundamentally why we teach in certain ways we need to identify the fundamental ideas that underlie our teaching strategy and the components of teaching that seem to work best for us and our students. We need to be asking ourselves a series of questions:

• **What techniques have worked best for me in the past? How do I talk about my successes?**

• **What evidence do I cite when explaining my success in teaching (e.g. to the dean)?**

• **What three-to-five phrases best describe my personal teaching philosophy, and how do these match up with my students' capacities and desires?**

• **How do I refine my teaching methods to reflect these characteristics? Having identified our teaching successes, the issue shifts to how we might better support the factors that brought success in the first place. The answers may have nothing to do with technology. More likely, however, they will.**

THE SEVEN PRINCIPLES OF GOOD TEACHING

Over a decade ago, Arthur Chickering and Zelda Gamson enunciated "The Seven Principles for Good Practice in Undergraduate Education" (*AAHE Bulletin*, Washington, American Association for Higher Education, March 1987). This list, with nearly a million copies in circulation, is very likely the nation's best known statement of teaching principles. Although it is unlikely to match perfectly the teaching principles of any individual instructor, the list provides a useful typology for exploring ways in which computers might enhance each practice. The seven principles are:

1. Encourage contact between students and faculty.

2. Develop cooperation among students.

3. Encourage active learning.

4. Give Prompt feedback.

5. Emphasize time on task.

6. Communicate high expectations.

7. Respect diverse talents and ways of thinking.

• **Encouraging Contact Between Students and Faculty**

How best can more contact be encouraged? Things that come immediately to mind are longer office hours, arriving at class early and staying after class, becoming the adviser of a social organization, taking a field trip, requiring a mid-semester conference, phoning each student each week, etc. New tools made possible by the computer include weekly e-mails to a class, with a weekly follow-up note to each student; threaded conversations concerning discussion questions that are overseen by the professor; electronic shuttling of the multiple drafts of an assigned term paper; e-mailing a class about the professor's intention of attending a campus event & urging class members to get together for a discussion after the event; having students share who will be visiting the instructor during office hours; asking students to answer a question prior to or a follow up question after a lecture; and staying in touch with students after a course has been completed. When redesigning a course, we can expect that some non-computer and some computer-based techniques will be introduced. Reconsideration is catalyzed by the new computer tools. Once a re-evaluation occurs, both computer and non-computer-based techniques will be retained, altered, or abandoned.

• Developing Cooperation Among Students

Cooperation among students can be enhanced by the computer in many different ways. Small groups of students may be encouraged to "edit" each others' essays prior to submission for grading, or to participate in a threaded discussion. Students may be encouraged to react to a classmate's in-classroom performance by sending e-mail messages to the presenter. All students may be encouraged to build, and subsequently draw upon, data bases that are enriched not only by students of the current semester but also previous students. In a writing class, a team of students can be asked to create a site on the Web that profiles a special author.

• Encouraging Active Learning

Computers can be especially helpful in facilitating active learning. Virtual art and music can be created with less expense and with greater capacity to accommodate multiple iterations. In the sciences interactive simulations can be assigned. References cited in the syllabus can be kept current by providing hyperlinks in the syllabus. Communication with class members on a field trip can make the trip real even for those left behind. Demonstrations given in class can be videotaped and made available to students studying the material that evening.

• Giving Prompt Feedback

One of the primary virtues of computers is the support of prompt feedback. A roomful of students can send e-mail messages to another student who has just finished giving an in-class presentation. Professor and student can stay in touch when either one is out of town. Paper submission deadlines can be assigned for any hour and day. Materials distributed electronically can be hyperlinks to, for example, the day's weather. Students can submit one minute (or longer) reactions to a lecture, during the lecture. Students can be polled for understanding during a lecture. Grades can be returned to students as soon as the grades are ready, instead of waiting until class meets.

- **Emphasizing Time on Task**

A big difference enabled by computers is continuous dialogue. Dialogue relating to the course can occur continuously, not only the (say) three times during the week the class meets. By encouraging pre-class discussions, threaded conversations after class, and even continuing contact after the final exam; a professors can significantly increase the amount of time students spend on a course. Moreover, because the computer can overcome the necessity of both geographic proximity and simultaneity, lecture notes can be made available anyplace and anywhere, tutors and course advisors can be available at odd study hours, experiments can be repeated outside normal class hours.

- **Communicating High Expectations**

There are a number of ways computers can be employed in the communication of high expectations. The best student papers can be "published" on the Web. This semester's students can be given full access to the papers submitted by students from previous semesters, with the hint that "this semester" is expected to do even better. Mediocre work is more easily returned to students with suggestions about how it might be improved, and with a request for resubmission. Students can be shown that their challenge is to extend knowledge, not merely rediscover it.

- **Respecting Diverse Talents and Ways of Thinking**

The computer is ideally suited for customizing assignments and accommodating diverse ways of thinking. Timid students may feel more comfortable entering "virtual" conversations. Multimediaminded students can submit papers using multimedia. Students who learn mathematically can seek out on the Internet alternative presentations of a particular topic. A single paragraph of text that is richly hyperlinked can be directed toward the intermediate reader, yet the same paragraph may be meaningful for the expert who can follow each hyperlink to expanded points. Team projects facilitated by the computer can expose more students to the practice of working in team and thereby overcoming some blind spots within any member of the group. Online tutorials also individualize. The computer is an important means of customization!

CONCLUSION

The wonderful thing about the computer revolution is the boost it has given to thinking about how we teach and how we learn. Much like changing the academic calendar from a semester system to quarters or vice versa, changing the level of available technology leads to constructive rethinking. To date, most faculty who have taken the time to consider the new computer tools have not only decided to try them, they have kept using them. This, along with the strong affirmation by students and their supporters (e.g., parents), suggests that as even more digitized resources become available, the use of computers through campuses and communities will become routine.

CHAPTER 8

LESSONS LEARNED

"Success comes from choosing one of the sensible futures and avoid one of the unfortunate alternatives."

Successful strategic change is rarely the pursuit of the very best alternative in the most efficient way. Instead, most organizational change is focused meandering. Success comes from choosing one of the sensible futures and avoiding one of the unfortunate alternatives.

So far, in this volume, the spotlight has been upon the sensible futures. Since it is equally important to avoid unfortunate alternatives, this chapter highlights a set of lessons learned by the early adopters of universal computing. The list is the author's summary of a Best Practices Conference held at Wake Forest in May, 1998. Participants, who are the co-authors of this list, are from IBM (Diana Oblinger), California's Sonoma State University (Mark Resmer), North Dakota's Mayville State and Valley City State's (Ray Brown), the U.S. Air Force Academy (Larry Bryant), the University of Virginia (Irving Blythe), Yale University (Dan Updegrove), and Wake Forest (John Anderson, Jennifer Burg, Craig Runde). Other contributors to this list are Don Sargeant (University of Minnesota at Crookston) and, from Wake Forest, David Blyler, Jay Dominick, Lynda Goff, and Rhoda Channing.

• **Develop a Comprehensive Plan First, and Quickly Match It With a Multiyear Financial Plan**

First, decide upon academic priorities, then a year-by-year flow of dollars that can be made available, and then determine an affordable strategy. It does little good to have a wonderful network if no one can access it, or computers for all students if there is no capacity to support their use in the classroom. Big dollars are required. It is unreasonable to expect that the level of funding required can be achieved in a single year. Multiple year planning brings clarity to the need for recurring dollars, not only capital budgets. And, by planning ahead it is more likely that thinking will anticipate technological developments.

• Focus on Four or Five Basic Themes or Decision-Making Principles

With computers there is always a still better option: a better hard drive, a more robust network, longer hours for the help desk. Balancing each component of a system against the others requires disciplined decision making, which in turn necessitates the articulation of very clear and focused objectives. Is the primary emphasis on academic uses or administrative uses? If academic, is the emphasis on presentation, analysis, communication, or all of the above? How immediate is the need? Key questions must be identified and answered in order to achieve consistency within limited budgets.

• View the Computer as First of All a Communication Device

Recognize that the largest and most immediate gains from ubiquitous computing relate to increases in the quality and character of communication within the community; then make decisions with this benefit in mind. First efforts in faculty development should stress ways the computer can be used to augment communication, for these uses yield a high and quick return with relatively small investments of faculty effort. Later, the more ambitious portions of the faculty can pursue macro-media and other more sophisticated uses of the technology.

• Take a "Wholistic" View of Education

Learning occurs both within the degree-credit classroom and beyond it. The biggest change computers bring to classroom work is what occurs between classes, not during class. Lecture notes can be sent out in advance. Students can discuss an issue associated with their reading prior to class, and follow up with collaborations or questions to the professor after the class. Communication can be continuous, even extending beyond the final exam and after graduation. In addition to these changes in degree credit instruction, the computer allows more students to be more "connected" with more interest groups and subcommunities. And the computer provides another way to work around limitations such as dyslexia or shyness.

• Capitalize on the Capacity of Computers to Provide Different Learning Experiences for Different Students

By experiencing and testing, we know that particular students learn best through visualization, through collaboration, through recitation, etc. Similarly, we know that certain subjects are more easily taught through a particular technique or approach. Best practice suggests expanding the horizons of students and faculty to recognize "different strokes for different folks."

• Encourage Multiple Use

The fullest justification for ubiquitous computing comes when computers are meaningful used not only in classes but also administratively, as in registration and marketing. Similarly, the Web page designed for use in courses leads to a still higher level of efficiency if the same design is used by student organizations, faculty committees, and personal pages. Proficiency developed through one use transfers quickly to other uses.

• Use Multiple Channels for Faculty Advice

Different disciplines require very different services from a computer infrastructure. One person, no matter how knowledgeable, cannot adequately represent this diversity. For a system to serve the entire community and for advice to span both shorter and longer time lines, multiple faculty groups providing planning advice on the same and on different issues is essential.

• Put Students First

The temptation to provide hand-me-down and obsolete computers to students must be resisted. A communication system is no stronger than its weakest link. If computers are to be effectively used in education, especially in strengthening learning communities, students must have computers that are equal to faculty computers. If collaborative learning is to be emphasized, all parties in the collaboration, especially students, need comparable computers. As we recognize that our newest students are already sophisticated in the use of computers and accustomed to learning via videotapes and other multimedia, that our youngest students will face a more technology-dependent world; the case for placing our college community's best general purpose computer in the hands of our newest students becomes compelling. Fortunately, university funders (legislatures, donors, tuition payers) are more easily won over to universal computers when we emphasize that students must have modern computers and therefore faculty need comparable equipment, than vice-versa.

• **Resist the Temptation to Build Every Bell and Whistle into Each Administrative System**

The main thing is teaching and learning, not the support system. In most universities there is constant pressure to pursue marginal increases in the elegance of administrative systems. Decision makers must maintain constant vigilance to assure that campus computer systems are first and foremost designed to meet the educational and academic needs.

In colleges we talk about academic and administrative computing. Often the systems require very different capacities. Administrative systems, for example, usually require tighter security, and involve tasks that are more likely to be repeated again and again. Once a system is designed for one of the purposes (either academic or administrative), the options for the tandem systems become somewhat constrained. If possible (it is often not possible in public universities with extensive governmental reporting responsibilities), it is best to design a system that works academically and then develop an administrative system that is compatible with it, rather than vice-versa.

• **Provide a sense of ownership**

Faculty must feel that they have a role in setting policy, and that the choice to enhance teaching with technology is theirs to make. Students must view their computers are part of the intellectual capital that will be with them for the rest of their lives: "The difference between privately-held computers and public stations is the difference between owning a car and taking the bus."

- **Communicate Consistent Expectations**

Predictability is important. Faculty must know when, for example, the computer system will be able to support the use of video in instruction. They must know the threshold level of computing accessible to all their students. Administrative statements must be crisp and accurate. Broken expectations, nurtured by overly optimistic or careless predictions, will break the system.

- **Improve Communications Weekly: Rumors Fly Faster**

Computers and communication cut two ways. Computers accelerate communication among class members and through sub-communities. These same channels, however, allow rumors to move so rapidly that they quickly seem true. It is important to anticipate fast-flying rumors by developing in advance sound and regularized systems for communicating with all constituencies. Communities need to be alerted early and often to scheduled downtimes. Deans and other senior academic officials need to issue bulletins at least monthly on the status concerning the phase-in of a stronger computer system.

- **Spread the Gains From and Ownership of Innovation Throughout All Units**

Building large empires in computer centers as add ons to other administrative structures is politically naïve, educationally unsound, and financially expensive. New dollars required for upgraded systems should be spread through an institution's structure. This allows existing offices gently to migrate resources toward the new system, and it means that all organizations can benefit from the new venture. Moreover, by assuring department chairs that they will have adequate staff to take advantage of new computers, by assuring the library that it will have a role in electronic as well as print media, by involving the "telephone support unit" in the administering of a new system of communication, political support for the expenditures is more likely to be forthcoming.

- **Ensure Reliability and Sustainability**

Faculty and students will soon abandon the use of computers if the network is unreliable or if an orderly plan for updating and refreshing computing capacities isn't in place. Cars will not be used when the roads are not open, and computers won't be used when the network is inaccessible. Colleges (and their supporters, such as legislatures) must treat computers as regular operating expenses that require upgrading each year, not as one time capital costs.

• **Decide Clearly on Either a "Standard Computer for All Students" Strategy or a "Threshold Standard" Strategy Where Students May Upgrade According to Their Personal Needs, Preferences, and Financial Circumstances.**

Avoid in-between strategies. From the "standard computer for all students" come efficiencies in training (neighbors can teach each other), less downtime (neighbors can share computers and a small inventory of loaners can cover those days when the computer is in the repair shop), fewer incompatibilities when pursuing collaborative assignments, easier transfer between curricula, a smaller parts inventory, greater sharing of teaching methodologies, and simpler resale of used machines. The inefficiencies of standardization come from the uselessness of previously owned computers, the extra capacity supplied to most students who could function well with a less powerful machine, and the strain of using a computer that is barely adequate by students in majors (such as math and physics) where more machine would be appropriate.

• **Choose One of the Poles: Commodity Buy (of Computers) or a Special Relationship With a Single Vendor**

In-between strategies are less efficient and less cost-effective. In both instances, colleges should establish "preferred computers." Although the advantages of full standardization are sacrificed under the commodity buy strategy, price competition is encouraged, students feel they have more independence, and politicians will get less pressure from excluded vendors. On the other hand, by relating to a single vendor the college is able to share responsibility for the viability of the entire system and gain advantages comparable to those provided by a "general contractor" when constructing a new building.

- **Establish "Preferred Guidelines"**

The university should identify a "preferred computer," a "preferred Web page design for courses," a "preferred software load," a "preferred basic classroom design, a "preferred refresh rate," and soon. These guidelines should be compatible with the emerging IMS standards for all courses offered from all countries over the Internet. Extraordinary support should be given to the preferred alternatives as an incentive for independent decision makers to choose the preferred option. An effective strategy is to standardize the computers provided to students, thereby building in a very strong incentive for faculty to opt for these same systems. However, it is essential in a university environment, where diversity is a basic strength, to allow faculty members with very strong convictions to deviate from the norm.

- **Recognize That the Economics of Refresh Rate Are Directly Related to the Rate of Technological Obsolesce. A Faster Pace of Obsolescence is a Strong Incentive for More Frequent Refreshing**

At the current rate of technological advance, if a student is provided one machine for four years, it will probably have much more power than is needed in the freshman year and be barely adequate at the time of graduation. Too much is paid for freshman-year computing and too little performance is purchased for the senior year. Three years seems to be the most reasonable cycle, although four years are possible if a very powerful computer is provided freshmen. One or two years is necessary if the university places a high premium on optimum performance.

- **Most Sunk Costs Can Be Ignored**

Computer processors become obsolete more quickly than automobiles. The costs of migrating data from one system to another can be daunting. It is often not possible for existing hardware to continue to support ever more sophisticated and complex programs. In the world of computing, it is important to anticipate the differential costs of upgrading old equipment versus the purchase of new equipment. The savage value of the old equipment must not be a major factor in decisions.

- **Purchase Equipment That Is Upgradeable, Both Computers and Servers**

Students need the flexibility to expand their computer's capacities when they enter a specialized major, or when there is a radical advance in basic technology.

- **Consider Leasing Computers**

This can include leasing all computers to the college or the leasing by vendors of computers directly to students. Most leasing contracts enable less investment up front, contain an escape clause that allows for a faster-than-anticipated refresh rate, and simplify the group purchase of software. When a university has the capital to purchase computers, the inventory taxes applicable to private-sector businesses can be avoided. In some states public universities have found that payments for lease are viewed as operating expenses, whereas purchases are treated as one-time capital expenses.

- **Calculate the Benefits and Costs of "Trickle Down" Assignment of Computers**

A few institutions have had success with assigning older computers to administrative users whose functional requirements are minimal. The economic gain from such practices must be calculated against the costs of transferring machines and of operating a system that includes a broader spectrum of models.

- **Utilize Strict Project Management and Don't Underestimate The Complexity**

It is important to have one person responsible for the overall management of the details of a massive computer upgrade project. Hundreds of independent projects, each preferably managed by different existing administrative units, need to be coordinated in terms of cost, personnel, and timelines.

- **Use a Hybrid Centralized and Decentralized Daily Computer Usage Support System (e.g., Help Desk Functions)**

Most colleges including Sonoma State and Wake Forest establish a pyramid of support that offers both decentralized consultants (e.g., one in each residence hall and each faculty building) and centralized consultation for more complex issues. Other campuses (e.g. VPI) reverse the pyramid. What seems most important is to establish a mixed or hybrid system so that weakness in one domain can be compensated for by strength in another.

• Provide Adequate Training and Help Desk Assistance

Universities must invest in training. Too often administrative effort focuses on getting computers into student hands. Assistance in use is essential. Both students and faculty tend to shun large learn-how-to-use-the-computer classes. Training programs that include "house calls" and "training on demand" tend to be the most successful. For example, it is more effective to train students how to use a particular software program at the moment they will use that program in a specific class.

• Rectify Quickly Minor Irritations That Are Not Costly to Fix

One of my favorites is the purchase of a $6,000 Super VGA Projector that was installed in a room that has no capacity for dimming the lights. By setting aside one-tenth of one percent of the total annual cost of computing into a make-faculty-happy fund, the distinctive needs (both real and imagined) of different disciplines and scholars can be accommodated without building for all departments and all students are overly expensive system. For example, if there are special programs needed by advanced physics students, it is cheaper to make those available only to the students and faculty who need them

• Stay Out of the Printer and Modem Business

Today printers are not much more expensive than a science textbook and are normally within the reach of individual students. The costs of printer ink, paper, and maintenance are exorbitant for public stations that are accessible twenty-four hours per day. Regarding modems, outsourcing Internet connectivity to commercial providers (such as AOL and IGN) is a cost-effective alternative to buying multiple lines and modems. Students who live in the residence halls and have access to a campus Ethernet system do not need to be provided any other means of Internet connectivity.

• Go Slow on Wiring Every Seat in Every Classroom and on Providing Every Classroom with Extensive Multimedia Capacities

The number of faculty who wish all students to use the computer during class is still quite limited, and the requirements for system reliability and system speed increase many times when all computers must be working simultaneously and all are trying to use the network in the same way at the same time. Although radio connections to the Internet are not yet sufficient robust for extensive in class use, the technology is moving rapidly and it is likely that robust radio systems will be available by the time there is a significant demand by faculty for all students to be connected to the network while in class.

• View Computerization of the Campus as a System, not as only the Computers Themselves

Providing computers to students is important, but it is only twenty-five percent of the expense and the work. Equal attention must be paid to network maintenance, reliable electricity, printing strategies, technical support in the departments, faculty development, and other areas. The system is as strong as its weakest link!

• Emphasize that Computers are a Means, not an End

CHAPTER 9

ANTICIPATING THE FUTURE

"15 hunches about the future"

The phenomenal rate of expansion in computing power per dollar and in traffic on the network will almost certainly continue for another five to ten years. Computers will become faster and cheaper. They will probably not become much bigger, because more and more computer tasks will be taken over by single-purpose machines and networks.

For me, the more interesting questions relate to the role and structure of societal institutions, especially colleges and universities and the communities in which they reside. How is this basic change in the technology of communication, storage, and indexing going to impact the institutions and traditions of our society?

This is the point where our futurists draw scenarios. They advance three or four equally probable visions for the future, each with the purpose of allowing us better to anticipate the future as it actually develops. By thinking about "what should we do if...?," we can greatly reduce the lead times required for response, even if the scenario turns out not to be fully accurate.

Scenarios are projections without the claim of clairvoyance. Through this set of fifteen ideas we offer one scenario that, though likely not to be fully true, will surely catalyze discussion and thereby give practice to decision makers for the future.

• Digitized Scholarship

The most authoritative and prestigious medium for scholarly publications will be refereed electronic "journals and books." Compared to printing on paper, electronic data are more interactive, sharable, searchable, linkable, revisable, updateable, and customizable. They are also more resilient, more cost-effective, and more diverse (e.g. movies and sound bits). "Publishers" will overcome the "migration problem" (i.e. old data unretrievable by new software) by maintaining data in multiple formats and reselling contemporary versions. (As a convenient secondary source, printed materials will continue to thrive.)

• **Humanities Scholarship in Teams**

The traditional humanities scholars will follow the lead of natural scientists by forming teams of researchers. The sole author tradition will fade. Driving this movement toward teams is the new need for scholars to seek co-authors who know computers, and collaborators who have access to digitized versions of the raw data. Interdisciplinary clusters of scholars, each of whom can bring distinctive methodologies and perspectives, can be identified, formed and nurtured even over long distances and across languages. Because all scholarship has become more accessible not only to students but also to scholars in other fields, increased pressures are developing to certify its soundness from multiple perspectives.

• **Farewell to Clear Disciplinary Boundaries**

Typical scholars will associate with a dozen or so affinity groups, some simultaneously and others sequentially. Large categorical labels, such as sociologists and physicists, are already poor predictors of the "set of basic concepts scholars share in common." With more sophisticated indexing and searching, temporary groups of scholars will fashion distinctive sets of common beliefs. Formed will be micro-disciplines. The large disciplinary categories, which have really been with us for no more than two centuries, will lose their meaning as each scholar sheds the unitary label and acquires multiple labels of the micro-disciplines. As a consequence, the disciplinary-departmental organizational structure of research universities will evolve toward the University of Chicago model of "committees of scholars." Professors will sell portions of their time to these committees, and it is with the committees that the doctoral students will associate.

• **New Typologies**

Today colleges and universities are variously grouped by geography, by level (2-year, 4-year, graduate professional), and by sponsorship (e.g., public, private, religious affiliation). "College graduate" is an umbrella concept that covers baccalaureate recipients from all types of institutions. Tomorrow, perhaps fifteen years from now, the diversity of experiences represented by the bachelor's degree will be too great for the umbrella. When the term, college graduate, is no longer differentiating, its use will diminish. New, more specific, labels will emerge such as "virtual college graduate," "residential college graduate," and "college graduate by test." The same colleges and universities will often be graduating all types. The use of the institutional categories of today will correspondingly diminish.

• Specialized Institutions

Seventy-five years ago, textbooks were a revolutionary means of providing all students access to the "lecture notes" of master teachers, often among the most respected members of their profession. In this new era, the textbooks will be "packages of text and video and sound and interactive conversations and linkages with authors." More than most textbooks, however, some of these packages will be capable of "standing alone" as a learning experience. Much like general merchandise and department stores, and much the general-purpose magazines such as Life and Look, all-purpose colleges and universities will increasingly share the "market" with specialty shops, shops which will not only offer programs of their own but also market many of their programs through existing universities.

• Collaborative Learning

Computers provide interactive technology. Students can be led to collaborate, when before geographic and scheduling rigidities limited the quantity and depth of group work. Out-of-class collaborations can be monitored by expert professors, who can intervene when appropriate. By combining theoretical learning and practice experience, the collaborative model is very powerful and likely to become as dominant in the 21st Century as the lecture model was dominant in 20th.

• Collaborative Teaching

Faculty can share their databases with their students. Departmental faculty can help each other prepare for class by sharing databases. Professional colleagues teaching the same course at several universities can divide responsibility for 32 class preparations, and thereby spend more time on the sessions assigned to them (which they share with students at other universities) and provide their own students interactive access to experts in each subspecialty. Cross cultural and comparative teaching becomes much more feasible. It is ironic that the same that gave birth to the textbook will also lead to its demise. Today's textbook attempts to provide the best "full set" of lecture notes to students in all settings. Tomorrow's "textbook" will be the loose confederations of materials selected by pre-eminent scholars of the "topic of the day." And, with inter-institutional bartering of time, students at many colleges will be able to hear, see, and speak with the expert who prepared that particular segment of the course.

• Hybrid Courses

Education is not about to become all "virtual." Few professors will subject their students to entire courses taught by new and untested methods. And, after testing, we shall certainly learn that some types of material and some types of individuals are "made for" virtual presentations, while others are not. All of this adds up to the practice that most courses will combine segments that are taught virtually and segments that are taught live. Even "distance learning" students will likely be gathered together in geographic clusters. And even fully residential students will be taking a course or two that is primarily delivered virtually.

• Guide by the Side

With increased degrees of freedom, increased access by students to data bases previously the domain of the professor, doubling of knowledge every several years and the resulting bafflement of information overload and, with the lack, at least currently of quality measures associated with information pulled off the Web; the role of professor as coach, motivator, sequencer, evaluator takes on new and expanded meaning. As the role for off-site and collaborative components expands, the strict lecture role for the professor diminishes. On residential campuses, we can expect class sizes to become more manageable and class time spent more intensively reacting to information gained before class rather than simply receiving information. The role of the professor truly becomes "the guide by the side" of each individual student.

• Globalization

The specialized institutions will be located throughout the world, not bound by local demand. Likewise students, now able to maintain electronic linkages with their home campuses, will find it easier to leave campus for a term or two. The world of education will grow smaller and more mutually dependent.

• Apprenticeships

In a fully digitized educational world, both students and faculty may stray farther from the traditional campus. Students may more easily combine classroom learning experiences with on-the-job training. Apprenticeships, already growing in popularity, are likely to become an essential part of virtually all educational programs.

• Corps of Professorial Associates

Practicing professionals no longer need to leave the locus of their practice in order to meaningful support the "book learning" phases of education. Very soon we can expect to see a professional school's graduates partnering with individual students. The one-afternoon "visiting MBA executive" lecture in business schools will evolve into a multi-year relationship which will be maintained electronically. College alumni will supplement professors' and college counselors' expertise by partnering with individual students. From our colleges will emerge the concept of "core faculty" and "associated faculty" that, unlike the adjunct faculty of today, are not limited by geography and the need for large blocks of time away from the job.

• Lifelong Relationships

It is obvious that the acquired dependency between the student learner and the infrastructure that supported the student while in college will be carried on to life-after-college. Increasingly students will demand access to the same resources, courses and technical support as they had in college. Students and professors will keep in touch more, much like the increased e-mail communication that is already occurring between college students and their parents. College alumni will continue to look to their school for educational opportunities, and the schools should look at how they can meet this interest before the demand is overwhelming. Similarly, there is a need to articulate the expectations of faculty and staff regarding continued contact with college graduates.

• Age of Experimentation

Many commentators have observed that the basic methods of teaching in college have changed little over the past two centuries. Because of this stability, there has been little experimentation with pedagogy in the academy. As a consequence, there has been little need for policies and practices that encourage, or even tolerate, such experimentation. This is, however, a new day. Where before there was a consensus among scholars about the best approaches to teaching and learning, today such consensus is non existent. We can expect this "age of experimentation" to last at least twenty years. Policies and practices within the academy must be adjusted.

• Age of Assessment

With experimentation will come assessment. Professors themselves will want to know what is working and what isn't. Society at large will want to know which resource investments are worthwhile and which are not. Metadata compiled from many institutions, over several years, will provide many new opportunities for analysis. The changes that take hold in the new era's educational community will be those that are demonstrably superior.

• More Communities

All scholars and all students will be more active members of more communities! These communities will be sustained for longer periods, even when the members are separated geographically. Lives will be rich indeed.

Afterword

An Invitation

The magic of universal computer access is the strengthening of interactive communities.

Our lists of metaphors, of lessons learned, and of "thinking ahead" ideas are meant to be a starting point. Please supplement and revise each of these lists with your own ideas. I plan to update each list on the first day of each quarter for the next two years.

Please send your ideas and thoughts in one of two ways. First, simply send e-mail to brown@wfu.edu. Second, if you would like your comment to become part of an ongoing conversation, post your comments at http://course.wfu.edu/intouch.nsf/($All)?OpenView. When prompted for name and password, use "wake" for name and "forest" for password (lower case and without quotation marks). After you've posted your comment, please tell me (by e-mail) that you've done so.

All who identify themselves with a posted comment will receive, at quarterly intervals for two years, an edited summary of key comments. By using one of our new tools to build a community, we can always be in touch!